AFTER ATKINS AND OTHER LOW-CARB DIETS

Lose weight and achieve optimum health with the Clayton Plan

Dr PAUL CLAYTON

ROBINSON
London

Constable & Robinson Ltd
3 The Lanchesters
162 Fulham Palace Road
London W6 9ER
www.constablerobinson.com

First published in the UK by Robinson,
an imprint of Constable & Robinson Ltd 2005

Publisher's Note: This book is not intended to be a substitute
for the medical advice of your personal physician. Always consult
a medical practitioner before changing your diet.

ISBN 1-84529-072-0

Printed and bound in the EU

2 4 6 8 10 9 7 5 3 1

Preface

This book is dedicated to my parents, who taught me the literal and lateral approaches to science; and to my children, who may still, one day, pick up the torch. I am indebted also to the many scientific and clinical investigators whose work I have borrowed from, and which is cited in this and in my other books. I have tried in this volume to make it accessible to a wider public, and incorporate it into a coherent whole.

There are few pieces of incontrovertible evidence in nutrition, few trials which cannot be criticised, refuted or re-interpreted. Much work in the field is under-funded, incomplete or imperfectly designed. Accordingly, and after studying many hundreds of scientific papers, I have tried to step back from the detail of individual studies to build what seems to me to be the most reasonable conclusions, from all the pieces of evidence, about the links between nutrition and health.

Some of the ideas developed in this book are fast becoming the new consensus. Others are still speculative. My aim is, first and foremost, to inform and empower the consumer. But this book is also a challenge to the scientific community to prove or disprove the pharmaco-nutritional approaches to weight and health management, all of which are easily testable, outlined in the following chapters. Finally, hopefully, it is a call to arms to those in the governmental and private sectors who could do so much more to improve the nation's health and well-being.

I would like to thank all the scientists, medeconomists, nutritionists, dieticians and other specialists who shared their time and thoughts with me during the writing of this book.

Contents

Part 4: New Directions in Total Health and Well-Being

Introduction: The Clayton Plan – A New Way to Health

In the last few decades our food chains have lengthened dramatic-ally, alienating many of us from the basics of food production and preparation. Over the same period there has been a well-documented series of food scares, and we have, collectively, become fatter – much fatter. Unsurprisingly, we have become paranoid about our food. Self-imposed dietary restrictions are prevalent, as are food allergies and sensitivities. Eating disorders in all their forms are now the norm, and we have become depress-ingly vulnerable to food fads and crank diets. In the face of overly complex problems many of us prefer to swallow easy, fast pseudo-answers than to face up to the real issues.

In the last few years low-carbohydrate diets have swept across the Western world. They have had such an impact that fashion-able US restaurants no longer serve bread at the start of the meal, and potatoes have become a taboo subject. But despite the popu-larity of the Atkins, Zone, South Beach and other versions of low-carb diets, our weight, collectively, continues to increase. There is, as yet, little hard evidence that any of these diets work in the long-term.

Despite this lack of supportive evidence, and despite growing warning signs that high-fat, high-protein diets may be actively harmful, low-carb has become a set of dietary rules for many. And this, in turn, has created a series of deep misunderstandings about the importance of different elements in food for total health and for disease prevention.

Quite apart from the aesthetic aspects, weight control is important for our health, but if we lose weight in the wrong way, we can end up doing more damage to our long-term health prospects than good.

Ideally, we should be able to combine long-term weight control *and* long-term positive health; health characterized not merely by the absence of disease but by energy, drive and an enhanced ability to achieve happiness.

The contemporary Western diet actively undermines this kind of positive health, and the low-carb diets are not much better. Try the next step: the Clayton Plan approach to weight and health control, which combines simple and delicious dietary schemes with comprehensive nutrient support programmes, to bring out and maintain the best in you.

How this Book will Change Your Life

This book will:

- explain why low-carb diets are not the answer to your weight and health problems
- tell you why you are likely to be overfed but under-nourished
- introduce you to the good carbohydrates that are low in calories but high in health benefits
- show you how you can eat to slow the ageing process and avoid many common illnesses and diseases
- provide you with an eating plan you can introduce easily into your life right now – a plan that will help you achieve optimum health *and* weight loss.

My aim in this book is both to dramatically improve your health and to help you achieve a healthier weight within weeks, but first let's take a closer look at the state of our health today and why we need a new approach to healthcare so desperately. You may well find the following alarming, but the facts speak for themselves.

The State We're In

The first thing that is clear is that excess weight is fast becoming our number one health problem. While the slimming industry grows fat – their profits increasing on a yearly basis – by offering us delusions of thinness, we are getting larger. In the last 25 years, obesity in England has increased four-fold from 5% to 22% of the population, and is projected to engulf one in four of us by 2010.[1] The figures are similar in most other Western countries. Fad diets come and go, but hardly leave a trace, and the impact of our increasing size, which spills over into increased risks of heart disease, diabetes, cancer, renal failure and other unpleasant diseases, already generates health costs of £7.4 billion per year. The message is very clear. The foods we eat are far from the diet we were designed to live on. The slimming industry has been unable to keep its promises.

But what about the state of our general health? How are we doing there?

The Shocking Truth

The facts about our state of health emerge in our actuarial tables – these are the tables drawn up by life insurance experts to determine premiums and the likelihood of insurance payouts. Life expectancy has increased by on average of two years per decade for the last half-century, largely due to public health measures, but our health expectancy has not kept pace. In 2001, British men could reasonably hope to make 75, while women scored a respectable 79.9. Unfortunately, men can expect to develop the first clinical signs of chronic degenerative illness at, on average, the age of 65, with women beginning to fall ill around four years later; so that both sexes experience a 'health gap', a period of increasing medical dependency, of around a decade.

To make matters worse, more of us are falling ill at ever-younger

Body Mass Index Table

Are You Overweight?

The Body Mass Index (BMI) is recognized as being the most effective way to check if you are overweight for your height. It is calculated by dividing your weight in kilos by your height in metres squared. A healthy BMI should be between 21 and 25. Check the table to see if you are within a healthy range.

Height	Healthy Weight Range (BMI 21–25)
5'0" / 1.52 m	7 st 5 lbs / 46.7 kg–8 st 11 lbs / 55.8 kg
5'1" / 1.55 m	7 st 12 lbs / 50 kg–9 st 6 lbs / 59.9 kg
5'2" / 1.58 m	8 st 2 lbs / 51.7 kg–9 st 10 lbs / 61.7 kg
5'3" / 1.60 m	8 st 7 lbs / 54 kg–10 st 1 lbs / 64 kg
5'4" / 1.63 m	8 st 10 lbs / 55.3 kg–10 st 5 lbs / 65.8 kg
5'5" / 1.65 m	8 st 13 lbs / 56.7 kg–10 st 10 lbs / 68 kg
5'6" / 1.68 m	9 st 4 lbs / 59 kg–11 st 0 lbs / 69.9 kg
5'7" / 1.70 m	9 st 8 lbs / 60.8 kg–11 st 4 lbs / 71.7 kg
5'8" / 1.73 m	9 st 13 lbs/63 kg–11 st 11 lbs/74.8 kg
5'9" / 1.75 m	10 st 0 lbs / 64 kg–12 st 1 lbs / 76.6 kg
5'10" / 1.78 m	10 st 5 lbs / 65.8 kg–12 st 6 lbs / 79 kg
5'11" / 1.80 m	10 st 10 lbs / 68 kg–12 st 10 lbs / 80.7 kg
6'0" / 1.83 m	11 st 0 lbs / 69.8 kg–13 st 1 lbs / 83 kg
6'1" / 1.85 m	11 st 4 lbs / 71.7 kg–13 st 7 lbs / 85.7 kg
6'2" / 1.88 m	11 st 9 lbs / 74 kg–13 st 12 lbs / 88 kg
6'3" / 1.90 m	11 st 13 lbs / 76 kg–14 st 5 lbs / 91 kg
6'4" / 1.93 m	12 st 5 lbs / 78.4 kg–14 st 8 lbs / 93 kg

ages. Once uncommon, asthma and allergy in adults and especially in children have increased dramatically. According to the University of Maryland, the prevalence of asthma has increased by 60% in America since the early 1980s, and has doubled in Europe. Australia and New Zealand have amongst the highest rates in the world. The lifetime risk of breast cancer in women was

1 in 36 when I was at medical school in the 1970s and 1980s (before switching to science), but has now reached 1 in 9.[2] Data from Cancer Research UK shows that the incidence of cancer overall increased by a third in the last two decades alone: from 30% of the population in 1981 to 40% by 1996. The incidence of cancer in teenagers and young adults has risen each year by around 1.2% per annum over the last 25 years, with the biggest increase among 20 to 24 year olds, where cancer is now the second leading cause of death (after accidents). Age-related macular degeneration of the eye, once a disease of old age, is now commonly diagnosed in middle-aged subjects[3] – and there are plenty of other examples of increased disease and accelerated ageing, from autism at one end of the age spectrum to Alzheimer's at the other.

To make matters worse yet there is a developing epidemic of Type 2 diabetes, no longer called adult-onset diabetes as it now affects so many young adults and adolescents. The disease is on the increase worldwide. According to figures provided by the British Diabetes Association and related groups, this condition may affect anything between 5 and 8 million Britons by the year 2010. This disease of our time, closely linked to weight gain, insufficient exercise and a poor diet, is coming to be regarded as a form of accelerated ageing which brings forward the onset of vascular disease (including heart attacks and strokes), renal failure, peripheral nerve damage, impotence and blindness.

As a consequence, it is hardly surprising that the numbers of adults and children who describe themselves as chronically ill has risen from 21% in 1972 to 35% in 2002[4]; and that spending on healthcare has risen throughout every country in the Western world. In the UK it has increased from 3.9% of gross domestic product (GDP) in 1960 to around 7.3% in 2003, accounting for 17% of total public spending. The rate of increase is accelerating, due among other things to the increasing numbers of diabetics, and should hit 10% of GDP shortly after 2010 if current trends continue.

What is also clear is that we can't rely on miracle drugs, or 'magic bullets', to make us better. Pharmaceutical breakthroughs are getting fewer and farther between. We have many hundreds of specific and potent drugs – so potent, in fact, that illness caused by the side-effects of drugs is now one of the leading causes of death.[5] Yet, with the notable exception of the antibiotics, we have hardly any cures. Almost all the drugs we use are palliatives which soothe or suppress the symptoms of disease but are unable to cure the underlying condition, which generally continues to deteriorate.

Health and Happiness

But have the economic, technological and medical successes of the last century given us, at least, peace of mind? Hardly. . . According to the UK Office for National Statistics, around one in three of the population have mental health problems. A very small number, perhaps 2% of the population, are seen by psychiatrists, but millions live below the threshold of clinically definable mental illness in a state of unhappiness and insecurity. According to the World Health Organisation, the incidence of depression is doubling every ten years and will be, by 2020, the most pervasive illness in the world. The widening gulf between the shape we're in, and the shape we'd like to be, in an increasingly commercialized and objectified world, makes matters worse for many, as shown by the increasing incidence of eating disorders in both sexes.

Something is manifestly going wrong with our health, our psyche and our waistline. The support systems we rely on are clearly not helping – and are making our problems worse by ignoring their cause, and concentrating on the most superficial of symptoms. Our guns are pointing out to sea, but the enemy is coming overland.

A New Way to Health

There is an alternative strategy, one which focuses on the causes of illness, obesity and unhappiness, and offers a fundamentally curative model for these and many other health and life problems. This is the emerging science of pharmaco-nutrition, a new science now being developed and taught at an increasing number of universities and colleges. This is the science that underpins this book.

Pharmaco-nutrition is fundamentally different from pharmaceutical medicine. It does not suggest that there is a pill for every ill. Rather, it marries the old wisdom that we are what we eat, with the scientific disciplines of pharmacology, biochemistry and epidemiology, to produce novel diets and multiple micronutrient regimes that reconfigure the body, and its complex metabolic workings. No more of the 'magic bullets' that wound so many of us, but support systems, free of adverse effects and curative in a way that drugs, by definition, cannot be.

The foundations for this new science have already been laid, and published in many thousands of research papers. This book draws the research findings together and translates them into simple guidelines which you can use to improve your chances of staying younger, healthier and slimmer, for longer.

Pharmaco-nutrition is a large part of my life. I design clinical trials on nutritional therapies for leading clinical centres; I teach medical students and doctors in five countries the benefits of nutritional approaches to disease prevention and I am currently involved in a number of exciting research projects that should help to make the benefits of pharmaco-nutrition available to everyone.

How to Use this Book

I have structured this book into four parts.

Part 1, Atkins Examined, looks in detail at the low-carb approach to eating. I look at just how likely you are to lose weight following that approach, I examine the evidence for long-term weight loss, and I take a close look at the health implications of long-term adherence to this diet.

Part 2, The Clayton Plan, introduces you to my healthy eating alternative. I introduce you to the 'good carbs' that are low in calories but rich in health benefits. And I provide you with recipes and eating plans to allow you to put theory into practice, quickly and easily. I explain why additives are not necessarily the evil they have been made to seem, and that much of the ill-health that has been ascribed by some to pollutants and additives is actually not to do with what is in our food – but what is no longer there.

Part 3, Fighting Disease with the Clayton Plan, provides more detailed advice on how changes to nutrition can bring about dramatic improvements in your health and well-being.

Finally, **Part 4, New Directions in Total Health and Well-Being**, looks at exciting advances in other areas of health and well-being including new ideas on how to give up smoking, anti-ageing approaches and novel ways to burn fat.

Now read on and learn more about the science behind this nutritional approach, how you can slow the ageing process through dietary change and why a low-carb diet is not the way to lose weight. And if you want to get started immediately on a new way of living, try Clayton Plan Top Tip 1.

CLAYTON PLAN TOP TIP 1

Today: Try starting your day with a bowl of fresh mixed berries and a sprinkling of almonds or other nuts. Add yoghurt if you like, but avoid the 'low fat' brands which are generally stuffed with sugar. It is better to go natural, and add a sweetener such as aspartame or sucralose (Splenda) if the berries aren't sweet enough for you. This combo is low in carbs and calories, and high in micronutrients.

1

ATKINS EXAMINED

- Why fruit and vegetables are vital
- Discover the good carbs that won't lead to weight gain
- Why eating a protein-heavy diet isn't good for your health

1
Will I Lose Weight?

It is hardly coincidental that in the last few decades, as we have become persistently larger, dietary fads have come and gone faster than ever before. High-fibre, grapefruit, cabbage soup, fasting, food combining, meal replacements and many more have come and gone, and all the while, the average waistline has continued to expand. None of these miracle cures has been very effective – except, of course, as business strategies.

But then along came Dr Robert Atkins. The sensation of the age, for most dieters, has been the low-carb, high-protein and fat diets. These actually date back to the 1900s, but were recently made fashionable once again by Dr Atkins, with variants such as the South Beach and Zone diets arriving later on the scene.

But just what is the truth behind high-carb diets, low-carb diets, surges of insulin and the effect on your weight?

Blood Sugar Levels and the Great Glycaemic Index Debate

First the basics on carbohydrates – they are an essential part of our diet! We know that our bodies are designed to use carbohydrates because carbohydrates (along with fats and proteins) are readily and easily converted by the body into energy. And energy is, after all, basic to keeping us alive. Energy keeps our body at the right temperature, it keeps cells regenerating, it allows us to think effectively and, obviously, it allows us to be active – to walk, climb stairs, clean the car, run.

Many carbohydrates are converted into glucose via the digestive system. To keep our bodies functioning at optimum level we need to maintain a basic level of glucose in the bloodstream – we also use the term blood sugar to signify glucose. What we eat has a direct effect on blood sugar levels, and certain foods raise blood sugar levels more quickly than others. Atkins was right to identify refined carbohydrates as problem foods in this regard. The effect of foods on blood sugar is measured by the Glycaemic Index (GI) and its scale ranges from 0 to 100 where 100 generally represents pure glucose. White flour – the primary ingredient of most breads, biscuits and cakes – has a high GI rating (of around 70) with potatoes, white rice, pasta and most breakfast cereals scoring between 60 and 90. Surprisingly, refined sugar doesn't score quite so highly (GI = 60), as it combines glucose with fructose ('fruit sugar'), which has a lower GI.

Pure fructose, as in the product Fruisana, has a low GI of around 24, and because it is 50% sweeter than table sugar, the amounts needed to sweeten a food or beverage can be reduced, with both factors contributing to significant reductions in the GI of the prepared food. Fructose is the main sugar in pure honey, which has led some to claim that honey is a healthier sweetener than table sugar. Unfortunately, the GI values of commercial honeys may rise as high as 80, because many manufacturers add large amounts of the cheaper glucose to bulk it up.

When we eat a high-carb diet, every meal pours glucose into the bloodstream, which is why such a diet is often termed a high Glycaemic Impact or high-GI diet. Each sugar rush triggers a surge of insulin release from the pancreas. This in turn clears glucose from the blood, driving it into the liver where a small amount is stored as glycogen; into the muscles, where, in the averagely sedentary person, a small amount is used to fuel exercise; and into the fat stores, where most of the glucose surplus to requirements is stored as fat.

This is all textbook stuff; but Atkins goes further. He says that the modern high-carb diet, by producing surges of insulin, creates periods of low blood glucose ('transient hypoglycaemia') which lead to increased appetite, increased snacking and, inevitably, increased weight.

He goes on to say that when we switch to a low-carb, low-GI diet, the body rapidly runs out of stored carbohydrates and is forced to switch to burning fats to provide energy. And because a diet containing more fats and proteins make us feel full, and because insulin surges are smaller and further between, we do not feel as hungry and we eat less. And because we are burning fat, and not replacing it, we lose weight.

But there are major holes in the Atkins thesis. To begin with the classification of food simply according to their GI rating is increasingly being recognized by dietitians as simplistic. A new term is now gaining wider usage – the glycaemic load of our diet or GL. The term GL measures both the type of carbohydrate in a food (whether it releases glucose quickly or slowly) and the amount of carbohydrate in that food. The GL rating is determined by multiplying the GI value of a food by the grams of carbohydrate in it. This gives a more accurate indication of the overall impact that food will have on blood glucose levels as some foods release glucose quickly, but in fact contain very small amounts of carbohydrate. For example, watermelon has a relatively high GI rating of 72, but contains very small amounts of carbohydrate so its GL rating is very low – 4. This is true for many other fruits and vegetables. For a list of foods and their GL rating see Appendix 2. What emerges from this is that banning all fruit on the induction phase of the Atkins diet is truly unnecessary in terms of reducing your glucose load. And as I explain later, it can have serious consequences for your health.

Examining the Evidence

Regarding the efficacy of the Atkins diet for weight loss, the jury is still out, but the verdict looks more and more likely to be 'non-proven'. There is good evidence that the Atkins diet is in fact a calorie restriction diet, and that the early weight losses commonly reported by Atkins dieters are the same short-term losses of water and glycogen that occur with every low-calorie diet. These are irrelevant to long-term weight control – and so far, there is little evidence that Atkins dieters do any better than any other dieters in the long-term.

In 2003, a small trial (on 63 obese men and women) carried out by the Weight and Eating Disorders Program at the University of Pennsylvania reported that weight loss was significantly greater in Atkins dieters than in conventional dieters at three and six months, but that these differences disappeared by 12 months. This was confirmed in an influential review of low-carb diets published in the *Lancet* in September 2004.

According to Professor Arne Astrup and his colleagues at the RVA University in Copenhagen, 'There is no clear evidence that Atkins-style diets are better than any others for helping people stay slim over a period of 12 months.' Their report stated that although there was evidence of initial weight loss on a low-carb diet, the explanation for this might be due to the restriction of food choices on such a diet rather than the low amounts of carbohydrate eaten. The report presented evidence that weight loss was associated with only the duration of the diet and the restriction of the energy intake, not with carbohydrate restriction itself. In other words, any calorie-controlled diet can produce initial weight loss. The report also suggested that weight loss might be due to the satiety effect of the high protein content of the diet; the fact that you are more likely to feel full after eating a protein-heavy meal. Satiety is an important point and one I will explore later in this book. The fact is there is a class of carbohydrate that provides good satiety levels together with a low-calorie profile and important nutritional benefits. The report concluded, 'Scientifically, the most solid current recommendations for people who want to lose weight and keep weight off is a permanent switch to a diet reduced in calories and fat, in combination with physical activity.'

The Arne Astrup report also examined the safety of low-carb diets. It noted that constipation and headaches are frequently reported on these diets and that such symptoms can be explained by the reduced intake of fruit, vegetables and whole-grain bread and cereals. The report continued, 'Restricted intake of these foods is not commensurable with long-term nutritional adequacy, and might pose a second-line increased risk of cardiovascular disease and cancer.' I look at these issues in more detail in the next chapter.

High-Carb Diets Around the World

High-carb diets do not inevitably lead to weight gain. Atkins was an American, who was familiar with the American combination of (over)eating, empty calories and lack of exercise, and he wrote his books about this very limited experience. If you travel round the world, however, you will find many countries where people routinely eat a high-carb diet but are not overweight. For example, the Japanese, and the vast rural Chinese and Indian communities, eat a traditional high-carb diet (noodles, rice, breads, etc.) yet have a very low incidence of obesity – although, admittedly, the incidence of obesity rises alarmingly in city dwellers who lead less physically active lives, and who have increasing access to American fast-food franchises.

Most clinical experts take the view that a calorie is a calorie, no matter what form you take it in; if you ingest more calories than you burn you will gain weight, and if you burn more calories

The Traditional Chinese Diet

Our understanding of Chinese food has been skewed by Westernized Chinese restaurants. The traditional Chinese diet is chiefly based around plant foods, with only small amounts of fish and poultry. According to Colin Campbell, director of the Cornell-China-Oxford Project on Nutrition, Health and the Environment, animal foods comprise only 20% of the traditional Chinese diet. Rice is a dietary staple, breakfast might be congee, a thin rice porridge; lunch is rice with vegetables and small amounts of pork; and dinner consists of rice and perhaps four other dishes, vegetables, tofu and perhaps a little beef or pork. In parts of rural China where this kind of diet is still the norm, breast cancer and heart disease are uncommon, and Type 2 diabetes and osteoporosis are much less prevalent than in the West.

than you consume you will lose weight. Let's look at this in more detail.

How Much We Used to Eat

Medieval feasts were traditionally served in three courses. The first course included a soup, which was followed by a wide range of baked, roasted and boiled fish and meat dishes. To mark the end of the course guests would be served an elaborate 'sotelty', an edible scene or maquette sculpted in coloured marzipan or dough designed to demonstrate the artistry of the chef, and the wealth and great good taste of the host. After a brief pause for reflection and the loosening of belts, the second course would ensue along pretty much the same lines as the first. Once the guests had done the second course justice, the third course would be summoned. In other words, each course contained the equivalent of an extensive modern meal, and the medieval diners were putting away three complete dinners, one after another.

Clearly, even though such feasts were not everyday affairs, our ancestors were not calorie counters, but nor did they need to be. The upper classes, of course, were well stocked with labour-saving gadgets (known as 'servants'), but for the yeomanry and peasants, life was physically hard work. Up to the end of the nineteenth century, all the tasks we now delegate to machinery, from washing machines to food processors, were done by hand. And the work was physical, too. Blessed as we are to be living in the Golden Age of Bureaucracy, where a hard day's work might run the gamut from word-processing to spreadsheets to a motivational seminar, it is hard to imagine an time when almost everything had to be made, stored, processed, grown or nurtured by hand.

Calories versus Activity

Look around the world today, and you will still find many areas where people live subsistence lives, scratching a living from the soil with little if any machinery to assist them. Heavy manual work of this sort requires from 3,000 calories a day (women) to

4,000 calories (men). If that work is being done at low temperatures, add another 1,000 calories a day to maintain body heat. Factor in strenuous exercise, as with polar explorers who insist on walking, skiing or roller-skating across the ice caps, and energy requirements reach 6,000 calories a day and more. At these very high levels of energy expenditure the diet changes dramatically, as only fats and oils contain the calorific density needed, and even then it seems impossible not to lose weight. Even on a diet containing around a pound of lard and 6,000 calories a day, a recent exploration team recorded body weight losses of 10% and more during their arduous trek.

For most of us, life has become much less physical. Where clothes were once beaten on rocks at the water's edge or on washboards, and then wrung out by hand, there came a series of progressively more efficient labour-saving washing machines. My mother's first top-loader washed the clothes in one tub, after which the sodden and lead-heavy clothing had to be hauled out, dragged through a (hand) mangle, and thence into a centrifuge

Exercise and Burning Calories

You've heard it before but it remains true that one of the most effective ways to lose weight is by increasing your level of activity. Here's a quick guide to how many calories you'll expend by undertaking particular sports and activities.

Activity	Duration	Calories Expended
Swimming	20 minutes	170
Cycling, at 16 km (10 miles) per hour	1 hour	540
Walking, at 5 km (3 miles) per hour	1 hour	300
Tennis, game of singles	1 hour	420
Squash	30 minutes	300
Jogging, at 11 km (7 miles) per hour	1 hour	360

before it was carried out to the clothes line. How laborious, compared to the do-it-all washing machines on offer today! And who beats carpets any more? Or clears out and then makes up the coal fires every morning? This explains why energy requirements today are, on average, a mere 2,000 calories a day.

Our food intake has shrunk over the past decades to go some way towards addressing this shift in our level of activity, but by cutting our food intakes in half, we have at a stroke halved our intakes of many essential micronutrients. And we still can't cut back our intake sufficiently to prevent weight gain – we are still taking in more calories than we are expending.

Muscle Power

We have been seduced by cheap energy and high technology, a sapping combination which has reduced our need to physically exert ourselves in many small and some not so small ways. Our bodies have changed physically; judged by the size of muscle attachment sites on bone, the working women of 200 years ago had better developed musculature than the salary-men of today.

This in turn has changed our chemistry and our health prospects, because muscle has metabolic effects as well as physical ones. Under normal circumstances (i.e. in 'normally active' humans), muscle is constantly in use so that if there is any excess glucose in the bloodstream it can always be cleared out of the blood (where you don't want it), and into the muscle where it will be put to good purpose. Active muscle is an active tissue – it uses glucose as a fuel. In this sense (and only in this sense) the muscle acts as a glucose sink. But because of the sedentary way we live, the volume and functionality of our skeletal muscle is compromised. This is one of several factors that impair insulin sensitivity, and are driving the current epidemic of Type 2 diabetes.

These trends led the World Health Organization (WHO) to declare, in 2003, that 'Lack of physical activity is already a global health hazard and is a prevalent and rapidly increasing problem in both developed and developing countries.' Only a year later, the WHO and the Food and Agriculture Organization (FAO) issued a joint expert report saying that 'Globally, overweight and obesity are now a more important cause of ill health than the problems caused by under-nutrition.'

How Many Calories Should We Be Consuming

When people's energy requirements have dropped to around 2,000 calories a day, as ours have, the complex regulatory mechanisms that determine our appetite find it very hard to keep up. Two thousand calories per day is not, after all, very much food, and at these low levels of food intake – and surrounded as we are by the siren songs of the advertising industry telling us to eat this, drink that – it is not surprising at all that it has become so hard to keep our waistlines in check.

How to Eat Over 2,000 Calories a Day

It's been calculated that most of us need to eat just 2,000 calories a day given the level of activity we undertake. But it's alarmingly easy to eat 2,000 calories or more in an average day – let's take a look at how that might break down for the average person:

Breakfast: 50 g (1¾ oz) cornflakes with dried fruit topping and 200 ml (7 fl oz) semi-skimmed milk, 2 slices of toast with jam and 2 teaspoon margarine; 200 ml fresh orange juice; 100 ml black coffee = 800 calories

Mid morning: 100 ml black coffee and 1 digestive biscuit = 170 calories

Lunch: Ham, cheese and tomato sandwich with butter, 100 ml blackcurrant juice, packet of crisps = 733 calories

Dinner: 1 cod fillet, grilled, 150g mashed potato, 50 g fried mushrooms, 50 g broccoli, boiled, 2 glasses of red wine, 2 digestive biscuits = 700

The grand total is 2,403 calories – significantly over the number of calories you actually need just to maintain your existing weight.

What's the Solution?

The success of any weight loss plan hinges not just on what we eat but how active we are. Exercise is a non-negotiable subject when it comes to losing weight. But so is your general nutrition. Remember, you are eating to keep yourself in optimum health. The biggest mistake the low-carb diet approach makes is to not pay sufficient attention to nutrition for the health of your body. By focusing on protein as a major dietary player, the low-carb approach omits the enormous health benefits of a wide range of foods.

More significantly still, the low-carb message has tarred all carbohydrates with the same brush. I want to introduce you in this book to the 'good carbs', a class of carbohydrates that are not only highly nutritious and provide good levels of satiety but which are also remarkably low in calories and have a low GI index.

The good carbs provide a truly revolutionary way of eating that will make your current daily obsession with the bathroom scales a thing of the past. More of them in later chapters.

CLAYTON PLAN TOP TIP 2

Today: Increase your activity – even the smallest change helps. Get off the bus one stop earlier, or walk or use public transport when you would normally drive.

2
Health Concerns

Despite the questions about the effectiveness of the low-carb diet for weight loss, there is widespread recognition that emphasizing or de-emphasizing the different types of food that provide your calorific intake might well exert positive or negative effects on your health. But here again, the effects of the low-carb diet are hotly disputed.

High density lipoproteins (HDL) or 'good' cholesterol can remove bad cholesterol from the linings of arteries and return it to the liver for processing and elimination. A small Pennsylvania study examining the Atkins diet found that the Atkins dieters raised levels of HDL cholesterol in their bloodstream by an average of 11% and reduced the level of triglycerides (linked to increased risks of heart disease) in their bloodstream by 17%. In the control group, the conventional dieters' HDL cholesterol increased by a mere 1.6% and their triglyceride levels were unaltered.[1] This suggested that the Atkins diet might reduce the risks of cardiovascular disease.

On the other hand, Dr Robert Eckel of the American Heart Association and many other cardiologists have said that the high content of saturated fat and animal protein in the Atkins diet would put people more at risk for heart disease,[2] and in 2004 Jody Gorran, a 53-year-old Florida businessman, sued Atkins Nutritionals and the Dr Atkins estate, claiming that the Atkins diet regimen caused him to develop severe heart disease necessitating surgery.

So do we go with Atkins or Eckel? Is the diet healthy or unhealthy? The reality is somewhat more complex; Atkins is neither implicitly good or bad, but may do good or harm depending on other aspects of the individual's diet, genetics and lifestyle. In order to determine the overall impact of the Atkins diet on health, we have to look at all of its major components, and the combined effect of their impact on the risk factors for heart disease and other forms of illness.

The Heart

From the heart disease perspective, it is possible to say with some conviction that the combination of increased intakes of saturated fats with reduced intakes of fruits and vegetables increases the risk of cardiovascular disease. This combination has been shown in many studies to increase the tendency of the arteries to become inflamed and constricted, a condition known as endothelial dysfunction.[3] This has been linked to a vastly enhanced risk of hypertension and vascular disease.

Set against this, there is good evidence that a diet which reduces the overall glycaemic load of the diet is cardioprotective, especially in people with raised glycosylated haemoglobin or HbA1c. HbA1c is a measure of blood sugar control in both the diabetic and the pre-diabetic, and is probably the most significant cardiovascular risk factor yet discovered. According to work done by Professor Kay-Tee Khaw at Cambridge and others, a single percentage point increase in HbA1c over the safety threshold of about 6% raises the risk of vascular accidents (heart attacks, strokes, retinal bleeds, etc.) by 10%. Conversely, a reduction of a single percentage point in HbA1c is predicted to reduce the risk of heart attacks and related episodes by 10%. Such a reduction can be achieved by cutting out a mere 30 g (1 oz) of carbs per day and, of course, the Atkins diet does somewhat better than that.

By these criteria, therefore, Atkins does rather well. In fact, if it were not for the more unbalanced aspects of the diet (the restriction of fruits and vegetables, the high amounts of saturated fats, and the poor design of the supplements), Atkins would probably be very cardio-protective, as well as effectively reducing the risk of developing Type 2 diabetes. On balance, however, in its currently undeveloped form it is probably neutral in its impact except, possibly, in individuals with specific lifestyle risk factors such as smokers, or with genetic risk factors, for example where blood levels of certain lipid fractions such as LDL cholesterol and triglycerides are unhealthily and abnormally high.

The Kidneys

A separate concern regarding Atkins is that the high-protein content of the diet is likely to increase the risks of renal failure. In 2003, a study which rang early warning bells was carried out at the Brigham and Women's Hospital in Boston, Massachusetts, and published in the prestigious *Annals of Medicine*. Dr Eric Knight and his colleagues followed 1,624 women aged between 42 and 68 over a period of 11 years, and found that 489 – approximately 1 in 3 – had a mild kidney problem.

The researchers found that in women who had healthy kidneys, there was no link between high-protein diets and a decline in renal function. But in those who already had a mild kidney problem, a high-protein diet, particularly one high in animal protein, generally led to a worsening of their condition.

Kidney disease is already very common, and becoming more so as the numbers of diabetics increase. And as the condition does not cause obvious symptoms until it is quite far advanced, there are increasing numbers of people eating low-carb, high-protein diets who are damaging their kidneys further without even knowing it. This means that if you already have pre-clinical diabetes (termed, variously, impaired glucose tolerance, metabolic syndrome or syndrome X), then low-carb, high-protein diets are probably not good for you at all.

Renal dialysis units are already in short supply, as are donor kidneys – another reason to treat low-carb, high-protein diets with care. The risks can probably be reduced by taking fairly simple precautions such as avoiding dehydration, and by using specific dietary regimes and supplements which can help to protect the kidneys. Avoiding dehydration is particularly important in elderly people, who often do not recognize cues such as thirst quite as effectively as younger people, and obese people, who oddly enough often confuse thirst with hunger and may prefer to eat when they actually need water.

The Bones

Concerns have been raised that low-carb diets may, over the long haul, increase the risks of developing osteoporosis.[4] This is due, it is claimed, to excessive acidity of the blood which can be caused by low-carb diets. This process is called metabolic acidosis. During this process increased amounts of calcium are lost in the urine. If other significant risk factors are present (such as early menopause, slight build, smoking, steroid use and so on), then the additional element of metabolic acidosis could well be significant. If none of the above apply, it is very likely that osteo-protective micronutrient support programmes will neutralize any increased risk associated with the low-carb regime.[5]

Fertility

Scientists recently warned that even a 'moderately' high-protein diet could reduce a woman's chances of becoming pregnant. High-protein diets similar to Atkins lead to increased levels of ammonia in the reproductive tract, but the significance of this was unknown until 2004, when scientists speaking at the annual conference of the European Society of Human Reproduction and Embryology reported that a diet containing 25% of protein significantly reduced fertility in mice.

The increased levels of ammonia disrupted the normal development of mice embryos at a very early stage in their development. The diet also affected subsequent embryo implantation in the womb and fetal development. 'Although our investigations were conducted in mice, our data may have implications for diet and reproduction in humans,' said Dr David Gardner, scientific director of the US-based Colorado Center for Reproductive Medicine, who led the research.

One cannot extrapolate directly from mice to men – or women. Nevertheless, this study sounds a warning bell, and raises a concern that will need to be more fully evaluated in further studies.

Cancer

Perhaps the most worrying of all the concerns raised in connection with low-carb diets arise from the evidence that high-fat, high-protein diets increase the risk of colorectal cancer. Even a 'normal' Western diet produces a stool which is carcinogenic[6] (contains significant levels of substances known to cause cancer), which helps to explain why colorectal cancer is one of the most common cancers in the West. On a low-carb, high-fat and protein diet, the degree of carcinogenicity increases, and this will, if unchecked, lead to an increased risk of bowel, liver and breast cancer in the long term.[7]

For the final word on diet and cancer I can do no better than refer you to the 1997 report 'Food, Nutrition and the Prevention of Cancer' published in 1997 by the World Cancer Research Fund in association with the American Institute for Cancer Research. Amongst the conclusions the report reaches are the following: 'The most effective ways of preventing colorectal cancer are consumption of diets high in vegetables and regular physical activity and low consumption of red and processed meat.' And regarding breast cancer, the report states: 'The panel notes that non-starch polysaccharides (fibre), regular physical activity, and carotenoids possibly decrease the risk of breast cancer, and that diets high in red meat, total fat, and animal/saturated fat, possibly increase risk.' And finally: 'Evidence of dietary protection against cancer is strongest and most consistent for diets high in vegetables and fruits.'

The Bottom Line

Reducing the amount of carbohydrate in the diet has received support from a number of nutritionists on health grounds. Walter Willett, Janette Brand-Miller at the University of Sydney and many others have also begun to attack the over-representation of carbohydrate foods in previous food pyramids. At the final maintenance stage of the Atkins programme most people are eating less carbohydrate than the 30% of calorific intake which is the current norm in the general population.

A consensus is beginning to emerge that the Western diet's characterization of carbs as being health-neutral is very wrong, as is our former characterization of the fats and oils as being intrinsically harmful. In other words, during all those years when fat was deemed to be the villain, and we agonized whether it was the butter or the margarine on our bread that was killing us, it was the bread all along. Atkins, therefore, saw a part of the puzzle correctly.

But where the Atkins and other low-carb diets fail is that they do not recognize the importance of the phytonutrients in fruit and vegetables; and they have not yet recognized the significance of all the research into different types of carbohydrates. Low-carb diets fail to take into account the most significant discovery in carbohydrate chemistry of the last fifty years, namely that there are basically two different kinds of carbohydrate. The old way of thinking about carbohydrates, in terms of 'fast' versus 'slow' or 'simple' versus 'complex' has been largely devalued. The new system of classification, which already has an extensive evidence base, differentiates between digestible carbohydrates and fermentable carbohydrates. I explain this in detail in Chapter 4, but first let's look at another crucial aspect of the low-carb diet – the severe reduction in eating fruit and vegetables, particularly in the induction phase. As I want to show you, the evidence for the benefits of eating fruit and vegetables is overwhelming – and the effect on your waistline is probably negligible.

CLAYTON PLAN TOP TIP 3

This evening: Try Chilli sans Carne (Chapter 7) for dinner. Chick peas and kidney beans are 'good carbs' – you will feel full and you will have boosted your digestive system.

3

But Fruit and Veg *Are* Good for You! Micronutrients for Super Health and Weight Control

One of the most controversial aspects of the Atkins diet is the severe reduction in the consumption of fruit and vegetables it requires. In Phase 1 of the programme fruit is banned altogether and vegetables restricted; in Phase 2 fruits begin to reappear but are placed towards the bottom of the 'carbohydrate ladder' in terms of the types of foods you should eat.

In this chapter I want to explain exactly why this flies in the face of so much evidence about the importance of these foods for our health, and why such a regime is not a healthy long-term dietary approach.

The Malnutrition of the West

Do you think you're malnourished? No doubt your answer is a resounding 'no, of course not'. Malnutrition is something we associate with dreadful TV images from the developing world – emaciated children with distended tummies or bone malformation. Malnutrition is the acute lack of calories that can kill within weeks or lead to diseases such as scurvy that result from the near absolute absence of an essential micronutrient. It is true that generally we don't suffer that type of malnutrition (called Type A) in the West, but I can virtually guarantee that if I conducted a clinical analysis of your diet, I would have to conclude that you suffer from Type B malnutrition.

Type B Malnutrition

Type B malnutrition is defined as a chronic depletion of micronutrients such as vitamins and minerals, essential fatty acids and other substances such as dietary fibre and the phytonutrients. There may be no obvious short-term effect from these deficiencies – although I would argue that many common complaints such as fatigue, depression and skin problems do result from multiple micronutrient depletion. However the most serious effects of Type B malnutrition are premature ageing and the early onset of chronic degenerative diseases.

How can we be malnourished, you might ask. We're eating plenty of food. In fact many of us are apparently eating too much food – or, at least, consuming more calories than we burn – and are overweight. The fact is that paradoxically, we do not eat enough food, and much of the food we do eat is 'micronutrient-lite'. Too many of the foods we eat today are overprocessed, contain the wrong balance of proteins, fats and carbohydrates and are low in too many micronutrients. Factors such as soils (and therefore crops) depleted in essential trace elements, prolonged food storage and inappropriate cooking methods mean that the overwhelming majority of us find it virtually impossible to obtain from our diet all the micronutrients essential for optimum health. Let's look more closely at what's happening.

Your Dynamic Body

Very few of us – perhaps 1 in 10,000 – die of old age. The vast majority of us sicken and die prematurely, picked off by 'natural causes' long before our biological life span has run its course. Cell culture studies, and the small but growing proportion of individuals who live on healthily into their second century, indi-

cate that our true life span may lie somewhere between 110 and
120.

But why is such a long and healthy life such a rarity? Why do so
few of us live out our biological potential? In fact our bodies have
miraculous processes of renewal which ought to ensure optimum
health well into our middle years and beyond.

First, all living tissue is dynamic – that is, it is constantly repair-
ing and renewing itself. Skin cells are sloughed off and replaced
everyday; red blood cells last for around four months before they
wear out and new ones take their place; you grow a new skeleton
every ten years or so. This type of change is imperceptible and constant. Cartilage in the joints is eroded and regenerated; atheroma,
the fatty deposit lining your arteries and implicated in heart problems, is constantly deposited in the artery walls and is constantly
being removed; calories are taken into the body in food every day,
and every day they are transformed into heat, movement and all
the businesses of life.

Early Symptoms of Possible Micronutrient Depletion

Although symptoms of depletion in certain vitamins and minerals
can be hard to spot, certain early warning signs may be important.

Symptom	Possible Micronutrient Depletion
Cracking at corners of mouth	Iron, folic acid, vitamins B2 and B6
Recurrent mouth ulcers	Iron, folic acid, vitamin B12
Dry, cracked lips	Vitamin B2
Rough, red or pimply skin on thighs and arms	Vitamin B complex, vitamin E, essential fatty acids (EFAs)
Eczema, dry rough cracked skin	Zinc, EFAs
Brittle or split nails	Iron, zinc, EFAs

Second, the body has incredible powers of regeneration and renewal, forged in the evolutionary fires of human development. If that were not the case, we would not have survived as a species. Our joints would wear thin by the age of 20, our arteries would solidify by 30, and our brains would burn out by the age of 40. And for most of us, that is simply not the case.

But, third, it is equally true that as the years pass, these types of degenerative change eventually gather momentum, and emerge in increasing numbers of us as clinical disease. This trend is so commonplace as to be almost beyond questioning – but I think we need to ask why this pattern is so prevalent. Just what is so different about old age?

During the first 20 years of life we are dominated by the processes of growth and renewal. As we age, however, growth and renewal slow, and the forces of breakdown and decay accelerate. By the time we have reached our late 40s they are predominant. We are now typically storing more calories than we can use, and the majority of us begin to put on weight. Our ability to heal is compromised; wounds, for example, take longer to mend, and are more likely to become infected. In general, the rate at which we can rebuild and renew our tissues declines, and is overtaken by the processes of decay. Little by little, therefore, tissue damage begins to accumulate, rather like the slow erosion of a landscape, whether we are talking about the slow silting of an artery, the equally slow thinning of the cartilage in a hip or knee, or the silent dying of our brain cells. We grow slow, ill and fat, and by the time we emerge, blinking, into the sixth decade of life, five out of six of us have the symptoms of one or more of the degenerative diseases, and most of us are overweight.

A number of theories have been advanced to try to explain this shift. The theory of an accumulation of genetic damage leading to a failure of tissue renewal held sway for some time, until it was pointed out that many types of tissue breakdown are extremely active processes, and if the breakdown side of the health equation ran down at the same speed as the renewal side (which the genetic damage model implied), this would lead to a general slowing of both breakdown *and* renewal. This is not what we see.

An interesting new theory which explains the evidence rather more convincingly, in my view, is based on the concept of Type B malnutrition. The processes of growth and renewal depend on the presence in the body of a number of vital nutrients obtained from your diet. These are, broadly, the vitamins and minerals, or trace elements – such as vitamins C and D, and the minerals iron, calcium, magnesium and zinc. These micronutrients are essential to the processes of bodily healing, repair and maintenance.

Essential Vitamins for Growth and Renewal

The tables below show the key vitamins and minerals for health, together with good food sources. The Suggested Optimum Daily Amount is my recommendation for the optimum levels of these nutrients needed to maintain health. You'll notice it is often much higher than the recommended daily allowances (RDAs) drawn up by the US National Academy of Sciences. RDAs were designed to prevent deficiency disease, *not* to achieve optimum health. The US RDAs differ for men and women. In this table the amount is averaged except for iron.

Vitamin	Benefits	Food Sources	Suggested Optimum Daily Amount	US RDA
A	Healthy skin, antioxidant, aid to the immune system; night vision	Liver, carrots, watercress, cabbage, squash, sweet potato	1800 mcg	800 mcg
B1	Energy production, brain function, digestion	Watercress, squash, courgette, asparagus, peas, cauliflower, beans	10 mg	1.2 mg
B2	Energy production, healthy skin, hair and nails	Mushrooms, watercress, asparagus, mackerel, wheatgerm	10 mg	1.2 mg
B3 Niacin	Energy production, brain function, healthy skin	Tuna, chicken, salmon, mackerel, turkey, mushrooms, wholewheat	60 mg	15 mg

Essential Vitamins for Growth and Renewal *continued*				
Vitamin	Benefits	Food Sources	Suggested Optimum Daily Amount	US RDA
B6	Protein digestion, brain function, hormone production	Bananas, broccoli, red kidney, beans, Brussels sprouts	10 mg	1.3 mg
B12	Protein production	Sardines, oysters, cottage cheese, turkey	15 mcg	2.4 mcg
Folic acid	Essential during pregnancy for foetal development; brain and nerve function	Wheatgerm, spinach, broccoli, sprouts, asparagus, hazelnuts	450 mcg	400 mcg
C	Boosts immune system; anti-oxidant	Peppers, lemons, kiwi fruit, tomatoes, broccoli, watercress	550 mg	82 mg
D	Good bone health	Herrings, mackerel, salmon	15 mcg	5 mcg
E	Antioxidant, wound healing, healthy skin	Sunflower seeds, sesame seeds, wheatgerm	110 mg	15 mg
K	Controls blood clotting, bone regeneration	Cauliflower, Brussels sprouts	200 mcg	105 mcg

Essential Minerals and Other Nutrients for Growth and Renewal

Mineral	Benefits	Food Sources	Suggested Optimum Daily Amount	US RDA
Selenium	Antioxidant, boosts immune system	Tuna, oysters, herrings	185 mcg	55 mcg
Zinc	Healthy nervous system, hormonal health, energy	Oysters, lamb, pecan nuts, brazil nuts	20 mg	10 mg
Calcium	Healthy heart, healthy skin and bones	Swiss cheese, cheddar cheese, almonds	980 mg	1 g
Iron	Energy production	Pumpkin seeds, parsley, almonds	10 mg	18/8 mg women/men
Magnesium	Healthy bones and teeth, healthy nervous system, energy	Wheatgerm, almonds, cashew nuts, buckwheat flour	400 mg	370 mg
Chromium	Balances blood sugar levels	Brewer's yeast, wholemeal bread, rye bread	150 mcg	30 mcg
Copper	Important for controlling blood pressure and antioxidant activity	Avocados, apricots, sesame seeds	2.5 mg	0.9 mg
Manganese	Healthy bones, stabilizes blood sugar	Pineapple, blackberries, raspberries	2 mg	2.1 mg

The processes of breakdown and decay are held in check by many of the newly discovered phytonutrients such as lycopene, lutein, the sterols, the flavonoids and the fermentable starches (see below).

A perfectly healthy diet would provide optimal amounts of all these micronutrients, enough to keep the processes of repair and healing ahead of or in step with the processes of breakdown and decay. This would keep the processes of tissue wear and renewal in perfect balance. Unfortunately, a great deal of evidence has emerged showing that the majority of people in the Western world are depleted in both the micronutrients for growth and renewal, and those essential to slow the processes of decay. This is emerging as a likely common cause of most of the degenerative diseases, and a large part of the process of ageing as we know it.

Let's take a closer look at exactly what these micronutrients are and how they protect us.

Essential Micronutrients

Antioxidants

One key group of micronutrients that can protect us against long-term damage to cells and premature ageing is known as antioxidants. In fact, many of them are more than antioxidants, and have a range of critical health-related properties. For example, some are anti-inflammatory agents, important because most diseases have an inflammatory element. Some also have the ability to prevent the denaturation of proteins, a biochemical process centrally involved in the progression of diabetes, and some have important anti-cancer properties. The risk of heart disease, blindness, cancer, asthma, dementia and arthritis can all be reduced with these micronutrients, which include not only the classic antioxidant vitamins and minerals (such as selenium), but also the flavonoids and carotenoids (see page 37). No single micronutrient is sufficient – our bodies need combinations of micronutrients that work in harmony.

There are some antioxidants in animal foods, but cooking destroys the major antioxidants in meat, milk and eggs, whereas the antioxidants in fruit and vegetables are much more likely to survive the cooking process, although eating these raw or lightly cooked is the best way to preserve the health benefits. As a matter of interest for the weight conscious, it's also worth noting how low in calories most of the best food sources are.

Classic Antioxidants		
Vitamins and Minerals	**Best Food Source**	**Calories per 100 g**
Vitamin C	Yellow pepper	15
	Papaya	32
	Guava	66
	Orange	37
	Grapefruit	30
Beta carotene	Carrots	24
	Spinach	26
	Peach	33
	Sweet potato	120
Vitamin E	Wheatgerm oil	899
	Peanuts (plain)	564
	Sunflower seeds	582
Selenium	Brazil nuts, dried, unblanched	710
	Tuna, light, canned in oil, drained	189
	Beef, cooked	200
	Spaghetti with meat sauce	100–130
	Cod, cooked	96
	Turkey, light meat, roasted	170
	Beef chuck, lean only, roasted	180
	Chicken breast, meat only, roasted	170

Fabulous Flavonoids

Flavonoids are substances found in plants that can protect the
body against a wide range of diseases. Over 20,000 have now been
identified since they were first labelled collectively as vitamin P.
Their discoverer, Szent Gyorgyi, named them after paprika, a rich
source of these compounds (see page 120). The flavonoids are
now divided into approximately 12 sub-types, many of which have
profound antioxidant, anti-inflammatory and other health protective activities.

Food Sources of Some Flavonoids

Flavonoid	Best Food Source	Health Benefits
Quercitin	Red and yellow onions, shallots	Cardio-protective; antioxidant, anti-inflammatory
Procyanidins	Grapeseed, maritime pine bark (pycnogenol), haws, flowers and bark of hawthorn, most parts of the yarrow, leaves and buds of hazel tree	Useful for arthritic conditions, protect the arteries, antioxidant, anti-inflammatory
Elagic acid	Walnuts, blackberries, pecans	Antioxidant
Catechins	Green and black tea	Cardio-protective; cancer protection
Silymarin	Milk thistle	Liver protection
Curcuminoids	Turmeric	Anti-inflammatory cancer protection

Carotenoids

The carotenoids are powerful antioxidants. They can protect
against macular degeneration of the eye[1] and coronary artery
disease[2] and are thought to have particular cancer-fighting

properties.[3] They improve communications between cancer cells and normal cells and this is thought to force cancer cells to revert to normal behaviour. Good food sources include carrots, apricots and squashes. Beta carotene is the best known. Lycopene is a carotenoid found in tomatoes (although they should be cooked to ensure that the lycopene can be absorbed by the body). It is an anti-cancer agent[4] and powerful cardio-protectant.[5] Lutein is another carotenoid, found in kale and spinach. It protects against macular degeneration of the eye[6], and is also probably cardio-protective.[7]

Sulphur Compounds

Pungent and often bitter tasting compounds, these are found in brassicas, a family of plants that includes broccoli, cabbage, kale and the Brussels sprout, quite possibly one of the best things to come out of Brussels. These compounds have been strongly linked to a reduced risk of a variety of cancers.[8]

Sterols

Present in nuts, seeds and certain seafoods (such as scallops), these molecules are chemically related to cholesterol, but act very differently in the body. A number of studies have shown they can help to moderate or re-balance the immune system, which is why sterols are used to treat such conditions as asthma and the allergies, and rheumatoid arthritis.[9] In Southern Africa, they are increasingly used to support T-cell function in patients with HIV; early results are very promising.[10]

Phospholipids

These are molecules which contain fatty acids, and are the building blocks of cell membranes and HDL 'good' cholesterol particles. They are present in foods such as egg (yolk), wheatgerm and offal meats – formerly a human staple in the West, but now generally fed to our pets.

Fermentable Starches

The star of the show, these are the 'good carbs', highly nutritious yet low in calories. And the best food sources? Legumes and pulses. It's worth noting that legumes barely make the Atkins dietary list in Phases 1 or 2. These good carbs are so important I've given them their own chapter (Chapter 4).

Atkins and Nutrition

A glance at the list of food sources for these essential micronutrients quickly shows you how important fruit, vegetables, nuts and pulses are, precisely the food groups you severely restrict on a classic low-carb diet. Fish, chicken and red meat supply a small number of these nutrients as well, but many are simply not present in these foods. And, of course, normally we eat these foods cooked, and the cooking process can severely deplete the nutritional value. A fat and protein-oriented diet will not provide the nutritional profile you need for good health.

But Atkins does recommend supplements, you may reply, surely that will ensure I get the right nutritional profile. Unfortunately Atkins was no micronutritionist, and the supplement recommendations, though they go some way to compensating for a very skewed diet, are not well thought through and in some areas are completely inadequate. For example, the importance of vitamin K, resistant starch, flavonoids and sterols to a healthy diet is simply not recognized.

Moreover there is plenty of evidence about the benefits of whole foods for health, such as the importance of fibre for healthy digestive functioning. Supplements can support a healthy eating programme, but your starting point for good nutrition should be the whole foods you eat at every meal.

Health Effects of the Western Diet

People who are depleted in all the essential micronutrients and phytonutrients listed above are heading for trouble. Tissue renewal is down, tissue decay and breakdown are up; these people are now accumulating tissue damage, and heading towards clinical illness.

To make matters worse, Type B malnutrition generally worsens as we age. Older people often eat highly restricted diets due to such factors as dental problems, difficulties with swallowing, a deteriorating sense of taste and appetite, and often reduced finances. This explains why we become progressively more likely to become diseased as the years pass.

It also explains why the degenerative diseases, and indeed obesity, have such long latency periods. Coronary artery disease, Type 2 diabetes, cancer, Alzheimer's and osteoporosis do not occur overnight, although the first symptoms might. These are slowly progressing conditions, which develop for decades before symptoms finally emerge.

In other words, the majority of apparently healthy adults are, in reality, pre-ill. They contain, in their bodies, the growing seeds of the illness(es) which will eventually become overt. Fat is accumulating, arteries are beginning to silt up, bones and joints are thinning, brain cells are dying. This will lead inevitably, eventually, to obesity, a heart attack, osteoporotic fracture, or clinically confirmed dementia. By that very late stage, of course, once symptoms have begun to emerge, the ability of the current medical system to put things right is very limited and generally restricted to suppressing the symptoms of the disease.

Why Drugs Don't Work

Ignoring preventive health issues leads to a truly bizarre situation. It is as if we taught car mechanics to carry out crash repairs, but nothing of maintenance. It is an inheritance from the early successes of pharmaceutical medicine, the sulpha drugs and penicillins which cured infectious diseases (the dominant diseases of that time) and laid the foundations of the pharmaceutical industry of today. Unfortunately, they also created models of disease treatment which are no longer appropriate to the diseases which are important now – the degenerative diseases. Even more unfortunately, these ideas still underpin the ruinously expensive system of crisis-management medicine currently on offer. They hugely influence the medical curriculum, dominate medical post-qualification training, and determine the overwhelming bulk of clinical research.

Pharmaceutical models which developed from the concept of 'magic bullets' (drugs which kill micro-organisms but do not hurt the host), and the closely related idea of specificity (find a target unique to the bacterium, which does not occur in the host), are fine when dealing with an infectious illness. They are not the right tools, however, for dealing with a degenerative illness caused by adverse lifestyle factors, and consequently many metabolic imbalances, going subtly wrong over many years. The huge increases in obesity, diabetes, asthma, cancer, psychological disorders and other diseases, the recent declines in life expectancy reported in parts of the former Soviet Union, Italy and the UK, and the persistent failure of the pharmaceutical model to find cures for any of these problems, tells us that we need a new way of looking at health: one which takes lifestyle and nutritional factors into account.

Sadly, despite the fact that the majority of risk factors and protective factors for degenerative disease are nutritional, nutrition as a subject is almost absent from medical schools. And because micronutrients are generic (i.e. they are not owned by any one company), there is little commercial incentive to do the studies that would provide the levels of proof that are required, for example, in the licensing of new drugs.

Pharmaco-nutrition – the Answer

Luckily, this situation is beginning to change. Literally thousands of small-scale studies have begun to chart the detailed relationships between diet, micronutrition and health, and have recently given birth to the new science of pharmaco-nutrition.

Pharmaco-nutrition starts by analysing the multiple metabolic errors that drive, for example, coronary artery disease. It then cross-references these against the known nutritional benefits of particular food-derived compounds, and finally assembles a comprehensive micronutritional support programme that rectifies all the metabolic errors, or as many as can be identified. This is not a magic bullet, but a comprehensive, multiple-support programme. Using this approach the chemistry of the blood and the physiology of the blood vessel walls can be reconfigured in a way that effectively immunizes the owner against cardiovascular disease. If disease is present it can be forced to regress, as the processes that drive it are damped and the healing processes that clean and remodel the arterial beds are supported and strengthened.

In a more general sense, the pharmaco-nutritional approach teaches us that the pattern of decline that generally runs in parallel with ageing is not inevitable. Diseases we thought of as inherently progressive are not; atheroma can be made to shrink, worn joints can be rebuilt. These diseases are called degenerative because, in a typical patient on a typically Western diet, they do worsen with age. But to assume that because this is what we always see, this is the way things must be, is a serious error.

Pharmaco-nutrition provides a hugely significant shift in the way we think about, and treat, illness and the symptoms of ageing. I personally believe that pharmaco-nutrition will prove to be as effective in treating and curing the degenerative diseases as the antibiotics were in curing the bacterial illnesses. And if that sounds too radical for the average doctor, remind them how the antibiotics were initially scorned by many practitioners, who felt that the infectious diseases were both natural (they are), and untreatable (they clearly are not).

Pharmaco-nutrition and Weight Loss

The principles of tissue dynamism, and the slow emergence of problems driven by slight imbalances sustained over long periods of time, also give us new ways of looking at the problems of weight gain.

The changes in our eating habits which have gathered speed over the last half century have moved us away from a high micronutrient, high-fibre, low glycaemic load (GL, see page 12) and low energy density diet, which encourages us to feel full at the end of meals, towards a low micronutrient, low-fibre diet with an excessive GL and high energy density, which does not. When the fast food franchises, with their finely honed commercial instincts, introduced progressively larger portions, they made matters worse.

To make matters worse, cheap energy and new technologies have reduced our need to be physically active, so we burn fewer calories; cars, lifts and remote controls have cut our calorific requirements by nearly a third in the last generation alone. Bear with me while I re-make this fundamental point: diet as we may, it has become almost impossible not to consume a hundred or so calories per day more than we now need. One hundred calories is nothing. But that is 700 calories too many each week, 3,000 excess calories a month, 35,000 excess calories a year, and so, gradually, imperceptibly, we leave our slim, youthful bodies behind and accumulate the avoirdupois of middle age.

A pharmaco-nutritional perspective, however, shows us that the excess weight that so many of us gradually acquire can be persuaded, with time, to recede like the snows of winter. At the same time, pharmaco-nutritional programming can halt and reverse many of the other signs of ageing, and help to uncover the individual's true physical and mental potential.

CLAYTON PLAN TOP TIP 4

For lunch try a salad of watercress, baked pumpkin and feta cheese, and scatter some pumpkin seeds on top. You will be eating a meal rich in protective carotenoids, vitamin A, iron and antioxidants.

4
The Good Carbs

My biggest single concern with the low-carb phenomenon is the categorizing of all sugar and starch carbohydrates as problem foods. They are not intrinsically bad, but they do become a problem when you combine a high-carb diet with a low-exercise lifestyle. I have already explained that these carbohydrates are a natural form of body fuel, and if we were more active, efficiently burning this fuel before it becomes stored as fat, we would have no problems with overweight and obesity.

Even more critically, the low-carb phenomenon has also failed to recognize the major breakthrough in the classification of carbohydrates over the past few years – namely the identification of the fermentable carbohydrates and their importance for health, satiety and weight control.

This chapter is designed to rectify the balance – to explain just what these good carbs can do for you and to reveal just how low they are in calories.

Understanding Carbs

There are two main groupings of carbohydrates it is important to understand – digestible carbohydrates and fermentable carbohydrates.

Digestible carbohydrates include the 'simple carbs', sugars such as sucrose and glucose, and the 'complex carbs', the starches in foods such as bread and potatoes which are broken down by digestive enzymes in the small bowel into glucose. These foods all contain about 4 calories per gram; and they all contribute to the glycaemic load of the diet, or the total amount of glucose derived from the diet which pours into the bloodstream.

Many diet books have focused on how simple carbs deliver glucose to the bloodstream more quickly than complex carbs. The argument is that this difference can affect our energy levels and therefore our appetite. In fact worrying about simple versus complex carbs is something of a red herring. The fact that these foods deliver glucose at slightly different rates may be relevant to sports nutrition, but it makes little difference to our long-term health prospects. What is important is the overall glycaemic load of our diet. The glycaemic load of the modern diet has been calculated as being nearly ten times that of the Stone Age diet, the diet that in evolutionary terms our bodies are still designed for. This excessive glycaemic load is now widely regarded as a major cause of diabetes, heart disease and certain forms of cancer.

The Fermentable Carbs

The fermentable carbs are treated completely differently in the body from the digestible carbs, and have a number of distinct and highly desirable characteristics.

The Ideal Low-Calorie Food

Fermentable carbs are low in calories. Fermentable carbs which are entirely broken down in the body contribute up to two calories per gram, but others such as polydextrose ('Litesse'), which are not completely broken down, weigh in at a mere one calorie per gram. Litesse is the brand name for a fermentable starch produced by Danisco, which is beginning to be used in processed foods. It is popular with food manufacturers because it can be substituted for starch and fats – cutting calories and reducing the GI, while adding the health benefits typical of the fermentable carbs. Food labelling law, which is about ten years behind the science, still insists that Litesse and similar products be labelled as fibre.

Zero Glycaemic Impact

Unlike the digestible carbs, fermentable carbs resist digestion, are not broken down by our digestive enzymes into glucose, and therefore have no glycaemic impact whatsoever. This is one of the most important considerations for our health, as I've explained above, but there are many others.

Encouraging Good Bacteria

The fermentable carbs pass through the small intestine intact into the large bowel, where they act as a substrate or food for the health-promoting bacteria that live there: lactobacilli and bifidobacteria, the very same bacteria that we eat in probiotic yoghurts. This process of fermentation, which takes place in all healthy guts, gives the fermentable carbs their name. And when these carbohydrates are broken down by the bifidobacteria, the end product is not glucose but short chain fatty acids such as propionic acid and butyric acid which in turn have important health benefits.

As the good bacteria multiply they suppress many species of undesirable micro-organisms that also live in the gut, including disease-causing bacteria and candida. This is, in itself, a highly significant health benefit which has been shown to reduce the incidence and severity of food poisoning and irritable bowel syndrome (IBS), but there is more. The butyric acid produced by the bifidobacteria and lactobacilli has been identified as being an essential nutrient for the cells that line the colon, and a powerful chemo-protective compound that very significantly reduces the risk of colorectal cancer.[1] Via slightly different mechanisms, the improved bacterial metabolism in the gut has also been shown to reduce the risks of liver and breast cancer.[2]

If that was all that the fermentable carbohydrates did, they

would qualify as the most functional ingredients in food discovered to date – but there is still more.

Reducing the Glycaemic Effect of Other Foods

As fermentable carbs pass through the small intestine they slow
the absorption of glucose from any digestible carbs that are also
present in the food, reducing its GI and the subsequent insulin
surge.[3]

Aiding the Absorption of Minerals

As the fermentable carbs enter the large bowel, the improved bacterial metabolism they create there increases the absorption of the
important minerals – calcium and magnesium.

Helping You to Feel Full

Resistant starches and the other fermentable carbohydrates
provide bulk in the food, reduce its calorific density and thus
help provide feelings of satiety. At the same time, the propionic
acid produced in the colon during the fermentation process is
passed to the liver, where it triggers metabolic changes that have
also been linked to appetite reduction.[4]

Fermentable Carbs and the Atkins Diet

Fermentable carbs produce an overall improvement in bowel
function, and an overall improvement in calcium and magnesium uptake; the production of ammonia in the gut is cut back;
and the carcinogenicity of the stool is potentially reduced.[5]

In this way fermentable carbs neutralize the potentially
adverse effects of low-carb diets on the bones of at-risk individuals, reduce the load on the kidneys (especially if they are used
in place of animal protein) and reverse the potential cancer-
promoting problems that can otherwise be produced by the
low-carb, high-protein, high-fat diets. (See page 25)

In healthfood circles, the best-known of the fermentable carbohydrates are the fructo-oligosaccharides known as FOS, naturally found in vegetables such as chicory, leeks and asparagus. Unfortunately, although widely sold by supplement companies, and promoted by Atkins in his *Vitanutrient Solutions* book, these are among the least useful members of this class of nutrient. Due to the molecular structure of FOS it is broken down very rapidly in the bowel, in a reaction which takes place almost exclusively in the ascending colon. This doesn't help to protect against cancer, which typically develops at the very other end of the colon. To make matters worse, the rapidity of the reaction floods the bowel with hydrogen, methane and fluids, too often resulting in flatus and diarrhoea.

There are other fermentable carbohydrates with rather more extensive molecular structures which causes them to be fermented very much more slowly, so much so that the process of fermentation occurs throughout the large bowel. This group, which includes the resistant starches, offer real chemo-protection, and the slowness of the fermentation reaction means that they are socially acceptable.

Food Sources of Fermentable Carbs

The best natural sources of resistant starch include lentils and legumes, and it is no coincidence that in parts of the world where these foods are staples (such as North Africa), the incidence of heart disease and colorectal cancer is very much lower than it is in the US or the UK.

Our own diet used to contain very much higher levels of resistant starch than it does today, but food processing technology and dietary changes such as the reduction in our intake of pulses and legumes have cut our intakes by at least half in the last century alone. Experts in the field such as Professor Joan Slavin at the University of Minnesota, St Paul, have linked this fall in consumption to the dramatic increases in colorectal cancer that have occurred over the same period. They advocate that we should restore our intakes of resistant starch to, at the very least, pre-World War II levels of around 10 g per day, in order to normalize our gut functions.

Food Sources of Fermentable Carbs

Food Source	Percentage of Resistant Starch	Calories per 100 g
Legumes		
Great Northern beans	28	118
Frijole negro (Black) beans	26.9	116
Haricot (Navy) beans (bean usually used in baked beans)	25.9	335
Lentils	25.4	100
Red kidney beans	24.6	100
Split peas	24.5	310
Cereal grains		
Sorghum	36.1	342
Corn	25.2	65
Barley	18.2	354
Brown rice	14.8	141
White rice	14.1	138
Wheat (cream of)	13.6	50
Millet (raw)	12.6	378
Oats (porridge)	7.2	368

Fermentable Carbs and Food Manufacturers

By a fantastic coincidence, the food manufacturers have also fallen in love with resistant starch, but for totally different reasons. Unlike almost all of the digestible starches, resistant starch is rather resistant to absorbing moisture. Cornflakes are made of digestible starch, which is why they go soggy as soon as you bring the milk anywhere near them. For the same reason, biscuits go soft unless kept in an airtight container. Breakfast cereals made from resistant starch, however, stay deliciously crisp right up to the moment you're ready to eat them, and biscuits made with this marvellous material retain their bite for far longer. Even better, replacing digestible starch with resistant starch cuts the calories almost in half.

Resistant starch, therefore, combines a host of health benefits for the consumer with an interesting set of physical benefits for the producer. Food manufacturers are convinced that there will be a growing market for this valuable new dietary ingredient, and are hastening to increase the production of resistant starches from wheat, maize, rice and even citrus peel.

Fermentable Carbs – the Way Ahead

In short, fermentable carbohydrates are now recognized to be an extremely important component in the healthy diet. But because they have only recently been 'discovered' (they were previously considered to be a type of dietary fibre), their importance has not been understood by the low-carb gurus. And unfortunately, the traditional low-carbohydrate diets are inevitably low in fermentable carbohydrates, which explains why the low-carb dieter can have poor gut function and flora, is usually constipated, has bad breath due to the process of ketosis, and in the long term maybe at an increased risk of developing serious diseases (see pages 23–24). In many ways, therefore, a phamaco-nutritional revision of the low-carbohydrate diets allows us to design an updated and improved dietary regime. This upgrade from Atkins is low-calorie, does not induce insulin surges, does not endanger the kidneys or the bones, and is undoubtedly cardio- and chemo-protective. This is a diet which recaptures the essence and the basic proportions of the way we ate back when we were hunting and gathering; but cuts the calorie content in half, and brings the Stone Age diet into the twenty-first century.

In the following chapters we will construct the new diet, and show how it combines calorie control with a range of health benefits that improve both physical and mental well-being.

CLAYTON PLAN TOP TIP 5

Banish the potato from your diet but introduce beans and lentils. These are a healthy and low calorie accompaniment to meat dishes and other vegetables.

2
THE CLAYTON PLAN

- Are you overfed but undernourished?
- A new food pyramid for the twenty-first century
- Recipes for optimum health and weight loss

5
The Clayton Plan Step 1:
How to Eat

Of course low-carb diets are not the way most of us in the West eat today. In this chapter I take a closer look at why, if we eat an average Western diet, we are so depleted in essential nutrients and what the impact is on our health. And I look at why additives in our food are not so much the problem as what's been taken out of the food we're eating. Finally I show you how you can begin to make practical changes to the way you eat and what you buy to start to reap real rewards in terms of weight control and health.

The Way We Eat Today

Despite our modern lifestyles, and the availability of a wider range of foods than ever before, most of us eat rather conservatively. The supermarkets know that many of us generally make a high proportion of repeat purchases, staying with products and brands that we know and feel comfortable with. Next time you find yourself at the checkout, glance at the contents of your neighbour's shopping basket or trolley – you probably do anyway – and see for yourself how strange and limited most people's food choices actually are.

Another factor that has affected what we eat are the changes in the way we eat. The rather old-fashioned model of parents and children sitting down together to eat a meal that mother (rarely father) prepared from basic foodstuffs is more nostalgic memory than contemporary reality. Most meals consumed today are captive meals, eaten in canteens at work, school, hospital, university, army base and prison. Then come the ready-made and often pre-cooked meals made to microwave at home: takeaways, from sandwich to pizza via such culinary delicacies as burger, chips and deep-fried chicken; and, of course, the fantastic proliferation of confectionery, snack foods and soft drinks that has continued to gather speed over the last two decades. The first generation of consumers to be exposed to large amounts of processed foods was at the start of the industrial urban age, when longer working days made ready-made foods an easy if not essential option. This created a generation of young working class men who, when they volunteered to be slaughtered in the Boer War, were found to be severely malnourished. The government responded by promoting cooking lessons and the first healthy ready-made meal: fish and chips.

The family meal had many different functions. It was important in the socialization of children. How many times have you heard parents complaining that their offspring just don't seem to be able to behave in restaurants as well as those nice French children do? Is it really just a coincidence that the family meal still holds a substantial place in French social life? And it was important, too, in teaching children to learn and then adopt adult tastes. Many green vegetables contain substances such as sulphur compounds, which we now know confer considerable health benefits, but which have bitter and pungent notes that children do not naturally enjoy. The ritual of the Eating of the Greens was actually a way in which parents could wear down their children's resistance and persuade at least some of them, eventually, of the joys of kale, broccoli and even the Brussels sprout.

This breakdown in family eating is critical in influencing our children's eating habits, and these in turn greatly affect their subsequent food preferences throughout life. Human babies are born with an inherent liking for sweetness, and an inherent dislike of sour and bitter tasting foods. Within a year or so they naturally develop preferences for saltiness and umami (or savoury) flavours

Eat Your Greens

It's true – greens are good for you. The brassica family of vegetables are packed with sulphur compounds that have been strongly linked to a reduced risk of a variety of cancers. These vegetables are exceptionally low in calories too. Remember steaming is the best way to reap the nutritional benefits.

Vegetable	Health Benefits	Calories per 100 g
Broccoli	Antioxidant, cancer fighting	24
Brussels sprouts	Antioxidant, cancer fighting	35
Kale	High in B complex vitamins; high in bioflavonoids and lutein	28
Cabbage	Antioxidant, cancer fighting, boosts immune system; high in choline (B vitamin)	16

and, by around the age of eight, many begin to enjoy sour flavours, especially when combined with sweet. This particular flavour combination has been developed in certain 'sharp' confectionery products which, aimed squarely at the child market, are practically inedible for most adults.

The bitter notes in beer, coffee and many green vegetables are generally only acquired in adolescence, with a learning curve that is hugely affected by the desire to be seen to be doing adult things. If a liking for these kinds of flavours is not learned during this stage of life, it may be difficult to acquire subsequently.

In our time, the pattern of three square meals a day has largely disappeared, and in many family homes today the individual family members hardly eat together at all. Given the pressures of work and time, children often eat on their own, and increasingly not in any communal space but in their own bedrooms. Increasingly, too, and in an echo of tribal culture, they eat different foods from their parents; they graze on strangely shaped extruded clouds of maize or potato starch, with small print on the packaging that parents can no longer read without glasses – but which, when deciphered, reveals lists of ingredients which seem to bear little resemblance to food as they know it.

The Way We Should Eat

One of the most important things you can do for your own health and weight control and that of your family is to slow down your eating rituals. Rediscover the shared family meal, try to adjust your busy schedule to allow more time for eating and truly savouring what you do eat. Try the following practical ideas.

- Eat at the dinner table rather than in front of the television or computer. Studies have shown that people tend to eat smaller portions when they eat at the table. Television and computers are distracting and can encourage snacking. A meal at the table focuses attention on the activity of eating itself – food is better appreciated and savoured.
- Begin the meal whenever possible with a soup. These tend to be relatively low in calories, and help to reduce appetite during the later courses.
- Eating at the table also tends to encourage better digestion of food. Eating food quickly and without proper chewing can lead to upset stomachs and inadequate absorption of nutrients.
- A family meal allows you to monitor what the members of your family are actually eating. Remember children and elderly people have special dietary needs. In particular, elderly people may not be getting adequate levels of nutrients – see page 30 for more information.
- Be careful with ready-made meals. Many of these are much too high in salt and sugar and, in general, the more processed the food you eat the more likely it will have lost essential vitamins and minerals. Salads, stir-fries and baked fish meals are all quick cooking options using whole foods.

Now let's take a closer look at what's actually in the food we eat.

Are Additives the Enemy?

I am not against additives. Some of them are actually phyto-nutrients, such as the food colourant lycopene, derived from tomatoes, and strongly linked to a reduced risk of prostate cancer[1], or micronutrients such as vitamins C and E. These and others are added in order to preserve the many foods we eat which are no longer prepared in the home kitchen. Instead they are assembled far away and on a huge scale, and must survive long and bacterially hazardous supply lines as they are transported, warehoused and retailed, right up until the moment where we consume them.

It is also true that in almost all cases, the stringency of the regulations concerning additives are such that we know more about the safety of the additives used than the foods we put them in. But this hasn't stopped many consumers from developing an almost paranoid perspective on additives, which has been fuelled by activists, a small number of poorly designed studies, and the increasing numbers of children who have asthma or some other allergic condition, food intolerances or behavioural disorders.

It is quite natural for us to think that these and other problems might be due to the presence of some noxious additive or pesticide residue in our diet. If we could only identify it, remove it, and purify our child's environment, all would be well. And of course we want our children to be well. But can it really be true that the amazing rise in allergy, for example, is caused by additives?

The Allergy Epidemic

Let's start with the basics. The incidence of asthma and the allergies has effectively doubled every decade since the 1960s, and today, asthma and allergy are reckoned to affect about one in five of the population, and as many as one in three children. The vast majority of allergies are to pollens, fungal spores and the house dust mite, but certain foods can also trigger allergic reactions. Although accurate figures are hard to find, the following figures are provided by the American College of Allergy, Asthma and Immunology. The incidence of allergic reactions to foods in the general population is between 1.4% and 2%, and about 90% of these cases are due to eight foods, namely fish, shellfish, eggs, milk, soy, wheat, peanuts, and tree nuts such as walnuts and pecans. A further 9.8% are linked to citrus, strawberries, kiwi fruits and a range of other foods, leaving only 0.01 to 0.23% due to food additives. The maths says it all: people are approximately 500 times more likely to have an allergy to a food than to a food additive.

However, there remain a small number of individuals who are clearly sensitive to specific food additives. Sulphite, the best documented of these, has been shown to aggravate asthma in about 4% of people suffering from asthma,[2] with steroid-dependent asthmatics being the most vulnerable. The benzoate preservatives have been put forward as possible culprits in some individuals; but this is difficult to evaluate as the parent compound benzoic acid occurs in many fruits, sometimes at far higher levels than are allowed when the benzoates are used as additives.

Behavioural Problems

Some of the synthetic food colours, and especially the yellow food dye tartrazine, have been linked to behavioural difficulties in children. This started back in the 1970s when allergist Dr Ben Feingold published a series of papers suggesting that susceptible children can develop adverse behavioural reactions to food additives. In the intervening years, the Feingold Hypothesis has been supported by alarmed parents and educationalists who had noticed the increasing numbers of children with autism, dysphasia, dyspraxia, attention deficit hyperactivity disorder (ADHD) and other types of learning disorder which are now reported to affect one in five of the school population.

In reality, however, the figures do not stack up. Amounts of additives have been reduced in most foods since the 1970s and although there have been a few rather poorly designed tests in schools over the last decade, the emphasis in serious science has moved away from additives towards the idea that an imbalance of fatty acids in the diet is the main cause of developmental and behavioural problems.[3]

The fatty acid theory of ADHD also sheds some light on the rival theory that food additives are responsible. People with fatty-acid deficiencies are often sensitive to salicylates – and salicylates were the culprit in Dr Feingold's original work. As is so often the case, as science progresses we learn that something we thought was correct is not entirely wrong, but is revealed to be a part of a larger whole.

Chinese Restaurant Syndrome

Another example of our irrational fear of additives is the case of the Chinese Restaurant Syndrome. The symptoms reported by the victims (twitchy limbs and a hot flush reaction) were attributed to monosodium glutamate (MSG), a flavour enhancer used in some Chinese foods. When MSG was given to people who claimed to have experienced the Chinese Restaurant Syndrome under test conditions, however, they did not react. This was hardly surprising as MSG occurs naturally in soy sauce, anchovies, parmesan and other delicious foods in which it is the main flavour component. The syndrome, if we can dignify it with that term, was probably caused by a toxic mix of excess alcohol and ethnic prejudice.

So when we attempt to alleviate our parental anxieties by shielding our children from dangerous food additives, we should think again. The simple truth is that once again we have been looking in the wrong direction, our judgement and emotions biased by folk memories of times past when the adulteration of foods was widespread, and the adulterants used (from chalk to arsenic) were the cause of social scandal, the subject of heated debates in Parliament, and responsible for much illness and death.

Developing Food Safety

By the mid-nineteenth century the problems of adulteration and the laissez-faire attitude of the government had made the food chain extraordinarily dangerous. In 1858 the worst case of mass poisoning on record occurred in Bradford, involving adulterated sweets. The intention of the confectioners had been to extend the mix by adding plaster of paris, as 'normal', but they had mistakenly used arsenic, so that over 200 people were severely poisoned and 17 died. Moral outrage was expressed in newspapers and periodicals and this combined with a series of papers in the *Lancet* by the Analytical Sanitary Commission, put enormous pressure on the government to act, and resulted in the Adulteration of Food or Drink Act 1860.

This Act was the first to deal generally with the sale of food and drugs in a pure state by promoting analysis of goods. The Recital to the Act stated that the practices of adulteration 'were a fraud on Her Majesty's subjects and a great hurt to their health', and acknowledged that 'more effectual laws than before were required to repress the practice of adulterating articles of food and drink.'

Food Safety – the Good Old Days?

Historians have traditionally blamed higher urban death rates from the late eighteenth century on poor physical living conditions and lack of food. However, it seems very likely that the higher numbers of early deaths in towns in the nineteenth century were related to poisoning. In 1820, Dr Friedrich Accum's *Treatise on Adulterations of Food and Culinary Poisons* showed that much of the bread consumed in London contained huge amounts of alum, effectively an anti-nutrient. Rum and beer were routinely watered down and then, to compensate for the lack of alcohol, adulterated with the intoxicants strychnine and Cocculus Indicus (a dangerous poison containing picrotoxin), and the colourant ferrous sulphate. Pickles, bottled fruit, wine and preserves were doped with copper sulphate, mustard and snuff with lead chromate. Sugar, sugar confectionery and chocolate were adulterated with ground glass, copper carbonate, lead sulphate and bisulphate of mercury; lead oxide was used to colour Gloucester cheese, and gin was laced with turpentine, alum and sulphuric acid.

Subsequently, a series of increasingly stringent Acts and the development of more sophisticated food analytical techniques gradually cleaned up the food chain, so that by the early 1920s the problems of food adulteration had more or less been brought under control.

Although our foods today are systematically sampled and more rigorously and scrupulously screened than ever before, the shades of the Victorian experience still linger. More recently, suspicions about the integrity of the food chain were reinforced by episodes such as the trade war between the manufacturers of butter versus margarine, and by outbreaks of listeria in dairy products, salmonella in chickens and eggs, and the BSE scandal.

All of these episodes have left many of us concerned and unsure about the safety of our food, and much of this insecurity has focused on additives and pesticide residues. But it is not so much the minute and probably insignificant amounts of additives and residues in our food that are causing the health problems that are prevalent today, but what is no longer in the food.

How Well Nourished Are We?

What we eat today is in many cases so little, and so nutritionally depleted, that, as I outlined in Chapter 3, most of us have Type B malnutrition. And this, in turn, has left our metabolisms askew and more reactive than they should be to foods and to other substances that, only a generation ago, were eaten and used safely by everyone. I believe this is the explanation for the rise in allergies and food intolerances we've seen in recent years.

In the last years of the twentieth century and in the early years of the twenty-first, a modern form of laissez-faire has returned to haunt us. We allow food manufacturers and retailers to sell us nutritionally depleted, unhealthy food and, unaware of the negative impact this has on our long-term health, we allow our children to eat the same foods. We need a new health commission: a campaigning group of clinicians, clinical scientists and concerned consumers who will put the food chain back at the top of our agenda, and reclaim our health prospects from the drug industry which promises so much – yet achieves so little. And this is because the root cause of much of our illness is to do with lifestyle, and particularly our multi-depleted diet.

Are You Getting Enough Micronutrients?

The US Department of Agriculture's Continuing Survey of Food Intakes by Individuals, and their intermittent Nationwide Food Consumption Survey, the largest of their kind in the world, paint a pretty bleak picture. They reveal that although outright deficiency states hardly occur, the majority of citizens are depleted in many micronutrients, in the sense that they do not achieve the RDA of those micronutrients.

Vitamin Intakes – US Department of Agriculture Survey 1994–1996	
Vitamin	**Percentage of population depleted**
A	55
E	68
C	37
B1	32
B2	31
Niacin	27
B6	54
B4	34
B12	17

Some groups are more likely to be depleted than others. Elderly people and hospital patients are at high risk, as are poorer people, and many children. This is often related to other aspects of the diet: according to the Institute of Medicine's 2002 report *Dietary Reference Intakes for Macronutrients*, higher intakes of sugars are associated with a dramatic decrease in micronutrient intakes, especially calcium. Basically, anyone who fills themselves with high sugar content foods (confectionery, soft drinks, etc.), will have less of an appetite for fruits, vegetables and other foods which would have provided better nutrition.

However, anyone outside those high-risk groups should not be complacent. The reality is almost certainly worse than the table suggests because, in many cases, the optimal levels of a micronutrient which will support prolonged good health are significantly higher than the RDA, which is set at a level only high enough to prevent deficiency disease (see Chapter 3). If the table were to be redrawn showing the percentages of the population who do not receive optimal micronutritional support in their diet, they would mostly rise up into the mid to high 90s.

Lessons from Our Hunter-Gatherer Past

Another way of looking at this pattern of multiple micronutrient depletion is to compare micronutrient levels in the Western diet with those in a hunter-gatherer diet, presumably the nutritional mixture we were designed to run on. This kind of data is hard to quantify but can be estimated from such sources of information as the content of Neolithic midden heaps, the calorie yield of different types of terrain and anthropological studies of vestigial cultures.

This kind of analysis allows us to draw up the estimates below.

Micronutrient	Main Food Source	Drop in Intake since Stone Age (as a percentage)
Flavonoids	Fruits and vegetables	75%
Vitamin C	Citrus fruits and berries	50–60%
Omega 3 fatty acids	Seafood	50%
Methyl groups	Offal	95%
Carotenoids	Fruits and vegetables	40%
Resistant starches	Pulses and legumes	50%

The table shows that our intakes of most micronutrient groups have fallen considerably since the Neolithic period. In many cases they have fallen in the more recent past. In some cases this is due to changes in eating habits; as vegetable and whole grain foods have been gradually replaced with meat and dairy foods, a very common trend as income increases, our intakes of flavonoids and carotenoids have fallen. In other cases it is due to changes in food processing, for example, the shift from crude vegetable oils to refined oils has lead very directly to reduced intakes of sterols and phospholipids. Modern food storage and the length of food chains has reduced our intake of resistant starch and many antioxidants. The changing geography of crop growth also plays a role, as happened when we stopped importing winter wheat from Canada and changed to home-grown. As UK soils are low in selenium, this quickly resulted in a lower selenium intake.

In many cases this fall in micronutrient intake has been caused by the almost universal decline in our intake of fresh fruits and vegetables that has taken place since the 1950s. This does not augur well for our health – and there are further worrying signs that the fruits and vegetables we eat today do not contain the same concentrations of micronutrients that they used to.

The Nutritional Content of Our Food

For many years, the nutritional content of the food we eat has been carefully measured and published in a series of editions of the nutritionists' bible, McCance and Widdowson's *Composition of Foods*. It was recently noticed that the mineral content of a wide range of fruits and vegetables declined very substantially between the first edition, published in 1940, and the most recent edition, the sixth, published in 2002.

Some suggested that this was not a real decline but an artefact, caused by our modern and, it was claimed, more accurate measuring techniques. This theory was disproved when the older techniques were dusted off and found to produce the same lower values as the modern methods. Something else had to have caused the drop in mineral levels, and two plausible mechanisms have been identified.

Changes in Farming Practices

First, there has been an evolutionary change in the fruits and vegetables we eat, resulting from the use of intensive breeding programmes to produce higher yields and enhanced disease resistance. It may be that the new varieties simply aren't as good at accumulating minerals from the soil they are grown in. And second, agricultural techniques have changed. The routine use of deep ploughing and NPK (nitrogen, phosphorus and potassium) fertilizers has altered the micro-ecology of the soil in a way that many experts think has been damaging for the plants.

There is a particular group of micro-organisms in the soil called mycorrhiza (from myco = fungus and rhiza = root), which grow in very close association with the root systems of plants, in a relationship which is probably symbiotic. It has been suggested that these micro-organisms assist the plant roots to take up mineral salts from the soil. Recent work by Dr Neil Ward at the University of Surrey and by others at Wareham has shown that deep ploughing and the use of NPK fertilizers leads to a dramatic decline in the numbers of mycorrhiza, and a parallel decline in the mineral content of a number of food plants.

NPK fertilizers are used to promote crop yield, and have undoubtedly helped to improve agricultural productivity. But it now seems that while crop yield improves, its mineral content may be going in the opposite direction. And there have been other changes in the plant foods we eat, changes which have been caused by pressure from retailers and, to some extent, from consumers.

Stir-fry Vegetable Mixes and Fruit Salads

From the retailer's perspective, boosting profit margins by 'adding value' and cutting production costs is all important. This is why there is so much emphasis on selling us pre-packed fruit and vegetables, as opposed to unprepared produce.

Unfortunately, vitamin levels in fresh fruit decrease after they are picked, and particularly after they have been cut and exposed to air or sunlight. Much of the peeling and chopping of ready-prepared produce is now done abroad and the food then undergoes a long journey before reaching British supermarket shelves.

In 2004, Which? surveyed the fruit and vegetables sold in UK supermarkets, and found that many had vitamin C levels far below normal for unprepared produce. Asda sliced runner beans, for example, contained just 11% of the textbook level of vitamin C, and Marks & Spencer's fresh mango contained just 42%.[4]

Bitter-sweet Corn?

But there is worse to come. Have you noticed how sweet sweetcorn is lately? Or sugar snaps, French beans and mange tout? The varieties we eat today are much sweeter than the vegetables our parents ate, because the supermarkets – reacting, presumably to consumer demand – asked the growers for sweeter strains, the growers asked the seed companies, and the seed companies asked the plant breeders. Breeding programmes have produced corn, peas and beans sweeter than ever before, with less of the bitter taste elements you will still find in the older strains.

But this may not be entirely a good thing. If a plant has been programmed to produce high yields and lots of sugar, it may well have less energy left over to invest in a group of compounds called phyto-alexins.

Phenomenal Phyto-alexins

Phyto-alexins have various roles, but many of them act as defence compounds which plants make to defend themselves against infection or predation by insects. The same compounds that protect plants against environmental attack can also protect us against harmful external agents. The flavonoids, carotenoids, sulphur compounds and others are now recognized as important phytonutrients which offer major health benefits such as cardio-protection and cancer risk reduction.

At the Institute of Food Research at Norwich, Professor Ian Johnson and his colleagues have shown that certain phyto-alexins (the sulphur compounds) are responsible for the bitter tasting elements in many vegetables that confer cancer protection. It is precisely these taste elements that plant breeders have tried to minimize, in their attempts to make sweeter vegetables.

In a related series of enquiries, Professor Rune Blomhoff's research team at the University of Oslo has shown that intensively grown fruits and vegetables contain consistently lower levels of antioxidants than do wild or organic plants of the same sort. These findings too indicate that intensive agricultural techniques, coupled with modern plant breeding, may produce high yields of good-looking, sweet-tasting fruits and vegetables – but at the expense of the plants' phytonutrient content.

All these factors are making some contribution to the prevalence of Type B malnutrition, as shown above, and this in turn is generally contributing to ill health. In some cases, however, we can be more specific, by going back to the basic attributes of some of the key phytonutrients.

The Importance of Phtyonutrients

- The sterols found in nuts, seeds and certain seafoods are important nutrients for the immune system. They effectively boost T-cell activity (the cells which attack viruses and other foreign bodies) while damping B-cell activity; a useful effect which has lead to many clinicians and therapists to use these nutrients to treat such inflammatory diseases as asthma and other allergies, and rheumatoid arthritis.
- Some of the carotenoids (found in carrots, yellow peppers and pumpkin) are antioxidants which have the ability to target and protect certain sites in the body, and have the additional property of killing and/or normalizing cancer cells.
- Many of the sulphur compounds, found in broccoli, cabbage and kale, increase the levels of detoxifying enzymes in the liver and other tissues, which hasten the excretion of toxins and carcinogens from the body.

- The flavonoids (see page 36) are potent anti-inflammatory agents, antioxidants and anti-glycosylants (they protect proteins in the body from damaging glycosylation reactions).

It is very likely that declining intakes of flavonoids and sterols have increased our chances of developing inflammatory, allergic and auto-immune conditions (including asthma, food allergies, ulcerative colitis and multiple sclerosis) as well as endothelial dysfunction, a chronic inflammatory condition affecting the lining of our arteries which leads to atheroma and hypertension.

It is equally likely that our declining intakes of lutein, a carotenoid found in green leaf vegetables, has increased our chances of losing our sight as we age, via a condition known as macular degeneration.

And it is easy to believe that reduced levels of anti-glycosylant flavonoids in our diet contribute, along with the vastly increased glycaemic load of the modern diet, to higher levels of protein denaturation, cataract, kidney damage, and insulin resistance.

How to Maximize the Nutritional Content of Your Food

A comprehensive micronutrient support programme can help most people maximize their health. In particular specific conditions can be avoided or improved with supplements (see Chapters 9 and 10) where it may be difficult to get the right level of nutritional support from diet alone. However, good foods are the foundation of nutrition and it is important to try to find the best produce available. Here are some practical tips.

- Never buy ready cut beans, chopped vegetables or ready prepared stir-fry mixes. Tests have shown the nutritional levels of these important foods are dramatically reduced once they have been chopped. Buy whole foods as much as possible and chop them when you are ready to cook them.
- Washed and bagged lettuce leaves are not so good either. Not only is the nutritional content of the leaf compromised, the

produce has travelled a long way by the time it reaches you and has gone through a number of chemical washes and treatments to eradicate fungi and preserve its colour and appearance of freshness. Try Little Gem lettuce for a convenient salad green option. Bought whole, it is easily prepared and provides a slightly better nutritional profile than Iceberg lettuce.

- Buy fruit and vegetables in season. The further your produce has travelled the less fresh it will be, and the fresher the food the more nutrients it contains. Read packaging labels to check where your fruit and veg have come from.

- Buy organic if you feel strongly about this. Organic farming may in some cases have less environmental impact, and there is evidence that certain organic crops contain higher levels of some phytonutrients.

- Buy your produce from local greengrocers and farmers' markets rather than supermarkets. Farmers' markets often sell a wider variety of fruit and vegetables and may sell more traditional varieties no longer found in supermarkets.

- Grow your own! The ultimate in freshness and control of pesticides and herbicides.

You now know how to shop, how to prepare your food and how to eat it. The following chapter explains exactly what you should be eating.

CLAYTON PLAN TOP TIP 6

> **Apples are an excellent source of beneficial flavonoids, but *never* buy them ready cut and chopped or in a fruit salad mix. You will be missing out on vital nutrients. Always buy whole fruit.**

6
The Clayton Plan Step 2: What to Eat

We begin with a diet that will provide a sufficient range and levels of micronutrients, in a user-friendly number of calories, to save us from the many adverse effects of Type B malnutrition and overweight. To that we add a moderate exercise programme – not one that depends on expensive gym fees or a personal trainer, but something simple which can be made part of your lifestyle easily and inexpensively.

A Varied Diet

As a rule of thumb a good diet should be diverse. We have seen so many fad diets focusing on one food type or another, but as our understanding of the relationships between food and health deepens, a consensus is emerging that diversity is the key. Several studies have shown that eating a wider range of different foods is in itself linked to better health and increased life expectancy. The Japanese are a case in point. Where Westerners are recommended to eat a minimum of 30 different foods a week (and actually manage only 15 to 18), the Japanese eat on average 27 different foods *each day*. A wider range of foods auto-matically increases the number of micronutrients consumed, and this certainly one reason why the Japanese are less prone to the 'diseases of civilization' – diabetes, heart disease and cancer – than Europeans.

The Japanese Diet

The traditional Japanese diet is packed full of nutritional treasures. Various soy foods are consumed, such as natto, miso and, of course, tofu and other bean curd products. These are good sources of isoflavones, phytonutrients with a variety of health-promoting properties. Japanese people also eat a good deal of fish, including oily fish – which raises their intakes of the valuable omega 3 polyunsaturated fatty acids, needed for the body's metabolism to work properly. Green tea is another nutritional 'star' particularly rich in disease-fighting antioxidants. A wide variety of vegetables play an important role – bamboo shoots, aubergines, various mushrooms, sweet potato and Chinese cabbage. Rice is a staple food, so that the Japanese actually eat a medium to high-carb diet. It's interesting to note, pace Atkins, that Japanese people have amongst the highest rates of longevity in the world, and generally low rates of overweight and obesity.

Some American nutritionists have come to broadly similar conclusions about the importance of dietary variety, and now recommend that 20 different foods should be eaten each day. Unfortunately, if you choose the wrong foods, and at an average of 150 calories per portion, this can easily add up to 3,000 calories per day or more. This might be acceptable for the active adolescent but is excessive for most middle-aged, sedentary and professional people.

So where do we start? There is general agreement that we should all be eating more fruits and vegetables – but how many portions of fruits and vegetables should we be aiming for? And what sort of fruits and vegetables are we currently eating?

Potato Peril

First, it is important to note that the ubiquitous potato does not count as a 'vegetable' in nutritional terms no matter how it is diced, even though it is the UK's favourite. In fact, according to the National Diet and Nutrition Survey of 2000, the most commonly consumed foods in children and adolescents are, in order of decreasing frequency: bread, savoury snacks, crisps, chips, boiled potatoes, mashed potatoes, jacket potatoes, biscuits and chocolate confectionery. In other words, the potato comes in at positions 3, 4, 5, 6 and 7!

You might have thought that age brought nutritional wisdom, but the results of the 1998 Survey showed a similar pattern in the ageing and elderly. Among the free-range elderly tea is the first choice, followed by the potato, with white bread and biscuits at 3 and 4 respectively. Among the institutionalized elderly the potato comes first, followed by tea, buns, cakes and biscuits.

Does any of this matter? The answer must be a resounding yes, because evidence is growing that the humble spud, now so very prevalent in our diet, has become a health hazard far greater than the more notorious member of its family, the deadly nightshade.

The potato, a tuberous gift from the New World imported into Britain in the late sixteenth century, was initially greeted with suspicion and only gradually accepted in European cuisine. By 1770, however, the French military chemist Antoine Parmentier's study of the potato had won a contest to find a food 'capable of reducing the calamities of famine'. He served dinners at which all six courses were made of potatoes, which I am not sorry to have missed, and many French potato dishes bear his name to this day, although not le French fry.

Potatoes consist largely of digestible carbohydrate, and most potato dishes have a GI close to the theoretical maximum of 100. When eaten, potatoes pour large amounts of glucose into the bloodstream. This was reasonably well tolerated by peasants and manual labourers whose physically strenuous lives meant that they needed to burn substantial amounts of energy each day. They had well-exercised muscles into which excesses of glucose could be transferred. Towards the end of the eighteenth century, however, as the potato became a more dominant element in the European diet, reports show that Type 2 diabetes was beginning to become a problem.

Then came the industrial revolution. New milling techniques produced a fine-milled flour, which, unlike earlier coarse-ground flours had a high surface area which produced a GI as high as that of the potato. The glycaemic load of our diet increased again as the nineteenth century progressed, and the incidence of diabetes rose in parallel.

Refined sugar plays a role also – although not the central role that some have allocated to it. Consumption of refined sugar had been on the rise since the 1600s, but had not made such a massive contribution to the dietary GL as only relatively small amounts were consumed. By the early 1900s, however, individuals' sugar intakes had reached 15 kilos per year, and had trebled again by 2000, as sugar is now a cheap ingredient in many processed foods. This added to the metabolic stresses of bread and potatoes, and poured yet more glucose into the nation's bloodstream.

In our time, and on top of a diet with an absurdly high glycaemic load, the cheap energy, high-tech culture has left us so under-exercised that our muscles are no longer the effective glucose 'sinks' they were designed to be. At the same time other changes in our diet, primarily our reduced intakes of fruit, have depleted us in a number of essential co-factors such as the trace

Chromium and Flavonoids

Chromium is an important mineral chiefly found in apples, eggs, nuts and mushrooms. White flavonoids occur in many fruits and in tea. There is evidence that a diet depleted in chromium and flavonoids can lead to insulin resistance and the development of Type 2 diabetes. Worryingly, a number of studies have shown that the average Western diet is very low in both chromium and the flavonoids.

element chromium and the flavonoids. The end result is the epidemic of diabetes we see today; the sixth leading cause of death in the US, and seventh or eighth in the UK. (The uncertainty is due to the fact that deaths due to stroke, heart attacks, kidney failure and other pathologies are often hastened by diabetes, but this is not always known or recorded.)

In this context the potato is no longer a cheap cure for famine but a major cause of disease, and quite possibly, as significant a hazard to the health of the nation as the contemporary New World introduction of tobacco. So push the potato to the side of your plate, hold the bread and the sugar, and let's review the current recommendations for fruit and vegetables.

Best Choices in Fruit and Vegetables

The UK official line for the recommended intake of fruit and vegetables is still five a day, but this is actually rather low and reflects little more than what the Department of Health thinks they might, one day, be able to achieve if the wind stays fair. A more fundamental criticism of the National Health Service five-a-day guidelines is that they underestimate the importance of beans and other pulses such as kidney beans, lentils and chick peas, excellent sources of the 'good carbs'. These only count once a day in their scheme, however much is eaten, because the NHS is not yet aware of the importance of the resistant starches that they provide.

A more genuinely protective level of intake of fruits and vegetables was recently announced by the American National Cancer Institute who now urge all men to eat nine portions a day, with their irritating catch-phrase 'Eating 5 to 9 and Feeling Fine, Fruits and Vegetables Anytime!' The French government, not to be outdone, recommends ten portions a day, and it is noteworthy that this is not far from the current French average intake of seven portions.

When the French diet is analysed regionally, a pattern emerges which underlines the French government's position. Consumption of fruits and vegetables increases as you travel in Europe, and indeed within France, from north to south. While health trends in the north of France are not so very different from our own national (un)health, the Mediterranean diet, which is strongly associated with a reduced risk of most of the degenerative diseases, as well as slowed ageing, contains close to the magic ten portions.

Colour Coded Fruit and Veg

Dr Jim Joseph and his team at the US Department of Agriculture Human Nutrition Research Center on Aging at Tufts University, who have been studying the impact of fruit and vegetables on the body's oxidative status, go further in the analysis of beneficial fruit and vegetables. They believe that it is not only the amount of fruit and vegetables that is important, but that the type and especially the colour are equally critical.

This is because many of the plant compounds that we use in our own bodies as protectants, and which are strongly linked to improved health and longer life, have rather different roles in the plants themselves. These are the phyto-alexins (see page 66) which the plant uses for a number of different purposes. They are part of the plant's defence system against disease and predators, but many have a dual role as signalling compounds, and provide

Optimum Fruit and Vegetables to Eat by Colour

Colour	Fruit	Vegetable
Red	Strawberries, tomatoes, raspberries	Red bell peppers
Orange-yellow	Oranges, mangoes, grapefruit	Carrots, sweet potato, winter squash
Green	Kiwi fruit, avocado	Kale, broccoli
Blue-purple	Blueberries, Concord grapes, plums	Purple cabbage, aubergine

colour cues that attract pollinators such as the bees or seed dispersers such as birds. As a general rule, the deeper the colour of the fruit or vegetable, the higher the content of these valuable and health-promoting compounds.

The Tufts team therefore recommend that the fruits and vegetables we eat should be as intensely colourful as possible, and have drawn up guidelines based on the spectrum of colour in plant foods.

This is a very reasonable starting point, but by no means a complete diet so let's start to build on this healthy foundation, and construct a new food pyramid which takes all the latest research into account.

Nutritional Profile of the Clayton Plan

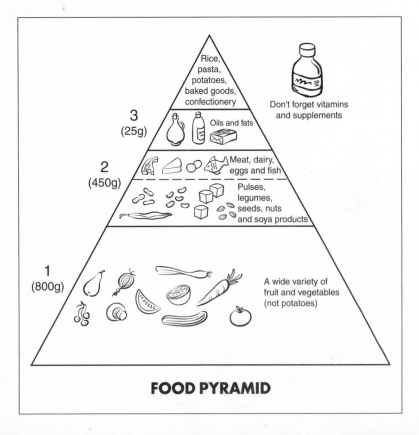

Rice, pasta, potatoes, baked goods, confectionery

Don't forget vitamins and supplements

3 (25g)

Oils and fats

2 (450g)

Meat, dairy, eggs and fish

Pulses, legumes, seeds, nuts and soya products

1 (800g)

A wide variety of fruit and vegetables (not potatoes)

FOOD PYRAMID

- The emphasis should be on eating a variety of fruits and vegetables, which form the first tier of the pyramid.
- Plant foods that combine resistant starch (lentils, beans and pulses) with protein (seeds, nuts and soy or Quorn products) and animal protein foods (meat, dairy, eggs and fish) form the second tier. The proportion of vegetables to animal foods should be about 2:1.
- The calorie-rich oils and fats constitute the third tier.
- Foods containing high levels of the digestible carbohydrates (potatoes, pasta, rice, baked products and confectionery) should be used only sparingly.
- For most people, a well-designed vitamin and mineral supplement is a sensible and desirable addition.

Calorie Breakdown of the Clayton Plan

The average energy yield of the first tier is around 0.5 calorie per gram. In the second tier the average energy content, brought down by the resistant carbohydrates, is around 3 calories per gram, while the third tier yields 9 calories per gram.

This means that a diet containing 800 g fruits and vegetables (equivalent to nine portions), plus 450 g of the protein and resistant starch foods, plus 25 g of the oils and fats, will still be under 2,000 calories a day. This mix provides a diet with a high micronutrient to calorie ratio (or high micronutrient density) together with bulk and fibre types which should satisfy most people's appetites. It also contains significant levels of the key protective and balancing elements, as would be expected in a diet that doubles the current WHO recommendation of 400 g of fruit and vegetables per day and it matches the levels of intake in the typical diet of traditional communities.

Protective Features of the Clayton Plan

- A key protective group in this pyramid are the resistant carbohydrates in the plant foods in the second tier of the pyramid, which protect against most of the potential hazards linked with a high protein intake.

- The preponderance of vegetable rather than animal protein in the second tier protects the kidneys.
- The phytonutrients in the fruits and vegetables at the base of the pyramid protect against the inflammatory effects that might otherwise be caused by a significant intake of meat and dairy foods.
- The bulking effects of the high intake of fruits and vegetables combine with the metabolic effects of the resistant carbs and the high plant protein content of the diet to help keep the appetite in check. At the same time they also help to keep the calorie count low, and the micronutrient density high.

This is a twenty-first-century version of the Neanderthal diet. It is probably very close to the dietary mix we were designed to run on, but crammed into fewer calories, in keeping with our less physical lifestyle. At the same time, if we start to build in the exercise programme, the calorie content of this blend of foods will start to promote a slow but sustained fall in body weight, and the gradual re-emergence of a much earlier body shape.

That might seem contrary to what we think of as the natural increase in weight that occurs in most of us as we age, but look around. Animals in the wild do not get fatter as they get older, nor do humans who live in traditional communities. And neither, despite our very different circumstances, do we have to succumb to the increasing waistlines that age usually brings.

Putting It All into Practice

Examples of the types of recipes and meals that will help you to achieve this are presented in Chapter 7, but here are some key principles to get you started:

- Snacks are not forbidden on the Clayton Plan. A morning and afternoon apple, pear, mandarin, or plum is a great way to boost your micronutrient intake, ensure you are eating the ideal nine portions, get an energy pick-me-up, and suffer no calorific overload.
- Reorienting your diet towards the fermentable carbs may need

some thought as traditionally Western cuisine does not feature these foods. However many other delicious cuisines do – for example, Indian cuisine features some fantastic lentil curries and bean dishes. Buying an Indian cookbook could be a very effective first step.

- Try to plan your eating plan for the whole day, remembering that lunchtime is a danger period when most of us during the week are buying food from takeaway outlets or in restaurants or canteens. One option is to prepare a curry or casserole at home and reheat this for lunch, another is to pack a salad. However, it's also possible, with some judicious shopping, to choose healthier options at the sandwich bar or restaurant. Remember to think vegetable rather than meat, fruit rather than chocolate or biscuit and search out the fermentable carbs wherever you see them – takeaway bean salads, for example.

- Remember that exercise can make an enormous difference to your total calorie intake – exercise burns the food you take in as fuel, muscles provide a sink for glucose. Above all exercise provides a host of other benefits from improving your cardio-vascular system to building strong bones and reducing the risk of several cancers.

Below I've provided some case studies to show you how to put my plan into action. David and Diane represent typical people with typical lifestyle and weight challenges.

Case Study: David, 45-year-old senior manager, height 1.80 m (5 ft 11 in), weight 85.7 kg (13 st 7 lb)

The Challenge

David's weight has been creeping up over the past ten years. Although he was a keen football player in his mid twenties, work and family commitments mean that he now spends less time exercising. He has a demanding job, involving a fair amount of client entertaining, and his lunches tend to be restaurant meals, often with a pint or two of beer. He's exhausted when he comes home and tends to wind down watching TV. In an effort to reduce weight he's taken to following a protein-oriented diet, but was alarmed by a recent health check, which measured his blood pressure as too high. His father died of heart disease in his early sixties and David is increasingly worried about his own health and weight problems.

The Solution
David needs a cardio-protective diet high in flavonoid-rich fruit and vegetables such as kale, broccoli, spinach, apples and cherries. Oat-based foods (such as porridge) and most types of bean can help reduce blood cholesterol levels and beans have good satiety levels, so that should help control his appetite. Subsituting soy products for meat will help and substituting red wine for beer will be beneficial. David needs to make time for regular exercise each day – to start with he could walk to the station rather than catching the bus as he normally does.

Sample Day
Breakfast: bowl of fresh fruit – chopped apples, cherries – a bowl of porridge and glass of orange juice
Mid morning snack: mandarin or other citrus fruit
Lunch: business lunch options could include Japanese-style miso soups, or Italian minestrone with a salad of tomatoes, cucumber, red pepper and lettuce
Afternoon snack: pear
Dinner: Baked Stuffed Mackerel with Leek and Lentils (see page 100)

Case Study: Diane, 38-year-old mother of two, height 1.63 m (5 ft 4 in), weight 70 kg (11 st)

The Challenge
Diane has found it difficult to lose weight since the birth of her last child five years ago. She is now back at work as a legal secre-

tary and finds herself exhausted each day with low levels of energy and tension headaches. She finds it hard to eat properly during the day, as she rushes from school run to work and then home again. She often eats later in the evening once the children are in bed and snacks to fill herself up. She had a recent health scare when her mother was diagnosed with osteoporosis and the specialist warned Diane that she, too, was at risk of the disease.

The Solution

Diane needs to eat more satisfying, but low-calorie, meals throughout the day and avoid late night snacking. She could switch to soy products rather than meat to obtain calcium and isoflavones; the green and blue cheeses are good sources of vitamin K_2, vital for bone health. Beans and tofu are good sources of magnesium and are also low in calories. Regular weight-bearing exercise builds stronger bones so Diane needs to incorporate this into her week. Exercising with the children could be a great way to combine her health needs with fun family time.

Sample Day

Breakfast: yoghurt with fresh fruit

Morning snack: apple

Lunch: salmon salad, fresh fruit, or bean salad

Dinner: Wild Salmon Oatcakes with Caper Sauce (see page 101)

CLAYTON PLAN TOP TIP 7

Remember weight loss is just part of your total health package. Any diet must also take into account other health risk factors.

7
Recipes

Diet books are depressing, and useless besides. It can be pretty demotivating to start a new diet on Sunday and have failed already by Monday evening, with nothing to show for your good intentions but cake crumbs and guilt. Luckily, this is no diet book. I am not trying to convince you to start a crash diet in order to reach your target weight in time for summer, because the figures tell us that that approach frankly doesn't work. Statistics don't lie, even if the diet gurus do. So, no needlessly complicated 'phases', no protein overload, and no recommendations to stop eating fruits and vegetables.

Healthy eating is different. It is a gradual change of diet, with the aim of re-educating your appetite and rebuilding your well-being. In the following recipes we show you how to use and combine ingredients that will reduce your calorie intake, increase your micronutrient intake, enhance your enjoyment of food *and* improve your health, all at the same time.

You might still fall off the wagon now and then. If you really need to splurge occasionally on something naughty but nice, enjoy it and don't feel guilty – because by committing to the kinds of recipes which follow, you will gradually re-educate your palate. The longer you stay with the new sorts of dishes in this chapter, the less you will crave the old ones.

As that happens, slowly but surely the weight will recede, and the scales will become irrelevant.

Basic Principles

Foods which can be eaten without restriction:

- fruits (except bananas and grapes due to their high GL)
- vegetables (except potatoes and swedes)
- beans
- pulses
- whole grain products
- vegetable proteins

Foods which can be eaten in moderation (3–7 portions per week):

- oily fish
- game
- dairy
- eggs
- nuts
- bananas
- grapes

Foods which should be eaten in relatively limited amounts (up to 3 portions per week):

- red meats
- pasta
- rice
- breakfast cereals (except those with a low GL value such as coarse mueslis and those made with resistant starch such as the Vogel's range)

Foods to be minimized (0–2 portions per week):

- confectionery (if made with sugar)
- soft drinks (if made with sugar)
- baked goods (except coarse breads, and breads and biscuits made with resistant starch – look for HiMaize, Litesse or, sometimes, resistant starch on the label)
- potatoes and potato products
- swedes

Exercise

Remember, exercise is vital for weight loss and general health. Aim for an exercise session at least three times a week for at least forty-five minutes on each occasion; preferably enough to raise a sweat and certainly enough to increase the pulse rate. At least two of these 'doses' of exercise should be load-bearing, i.e. not swimming.

Bon appetit!

> When flour is mentioned, use resistant starch if you can get it. If this is not possible, use gram (chickpea) flour, and other bean flours, which can be used in baking and have very low GL values. Low-sodium salt should also be used instead of ordinary salt.

Breakfast Options

I haven't included recipes for breakfast as the principles to follow for healthy eating are fairly straight forward. But remember, this really is one of the most important meals of the day for refuelling and activating your energy levels. Here are some general principles to follow:

- Fruits are a great way to start the day and increase your portions so you start to reach the recommended nine portions daily.
- Natural (unsweetened) yoghurts are also a good choice and can be sweetened with sucralose (Splenda), aspartame or fruit sugar as desired.
- Eggs are great, as are kippers.
- Most breakfast cereals are not such a good choice, but Vogel's cereals are good and oat-based products are OK *if* the oats are coarse crushed or rolled, which brings the GL down.
- Muesli products made from such oats are OK too, and if nuts and seeds are included, all the better, together with some dried fruit.
- Start with tea or coffee (which help to reduce appetite somewhat).

Starters or Lunches

Tuscan Bean Soup: Serving Size: 4–6

Ingredients

- 2 tablespoons extra virgin olive oil
- 1 large onion, chopped
- 6 cloves garlic, minced or crushed
- 845 ml/1½ pint vegetable broth, or 1 good vegetable stock cube
- 1 × 454 g/16 oz tin tomatoes (undrained), chopped
- 1 teaspoon dried basil (or 6 fresh leaves, if you have them)
- ½ teaspoon dried oregano
- 170 g/6 oz fresh parsley
- pepper to taste
- 1 teaspoon of tomato paste (optional)
- 1 × 454 g/16 oz tin cannellini beans, usually in salted water

Method

Drain and rinse the cannellini beans thoroughly.

Heat the olive oil in a large pan or casserole (with a lid) over medium heat. Add onion and sauté for about 1 minute. Add the garlic, broth, tomatoes, tomato paste, spices and parsley.

If using a stock cube, make up in 845 ml/1½ pint of boiled water, add stock to the pan. Bring to the boil, reduce heat to low and cover. Simmer for about 10 minutes, stirring occasionally, then remove from heat and blend thoroughly.

Add the beans, replace on low heat and simmer for at least 40 minutes. If you prefer a creamier consistency, use a blender or masher to break down the beans before serving.

Sag Daal: Serving Size: 2

Ingredients

- 340 g/12 oz green or red lentils, split peas or other pulse
- 454 g/16 oz spinach
- ½ teaspoon salt (low sodium salt is an option)
- ½ teaspoon turmeric
- ½ teaspoon medium chilli powder
- 2 tablespoons vegetable oil
- 1 onion, finely chopped
- 4 cloves garlic, finely chopped or crushed (optional)
- ½ teaspoon cumin seed
- 1 teaspoon mustard seed
- 1 teaspoon garam masala

Method

Wash the pulses and soak in water. In a large saucepan, put 845 ml/1½ pint of water on to boil. Wash, drain and chop the spinach finely.

When the water boils add the drained pulses, salt, turmeric and chilli powder. Return to the boil and cook for 5 minutes. Stir in the spinach and continue cooking over a medium heat.

Meanwhile, heat the oil in a frying pan. Fry the onion, garlic, cumin and mustard seed until the onions are golden. Stir this into the pulse and spinach mix. Add the garam masala.

Continue cooking over a low heat until the daal is soft and there is little excess water left. (If the dish gets too dry before serving, add a small quantity of water to bring it back to the right consistency.)

Aztec Three Bean Salad: Serving Size: 4

Ingredients

- 1 × 454 g/16 oz tin green beans
- 1 × 454 g/16 oz tin chick peas
- 1 × 454 g/16 oz tin kidney beans
- 1 green pepper, chopped
- ½ red onion, chopped
- 114 ml/4 fl oz cider vinegar
- 57 g/2 oz fruit sugar
- ½ teaspoon salt
- ½ teaspoon pepper
- 114 ml/4 fl oz corn oil
- 170–227 g/6–8 oz mixed leaves, e.g. lollo rosso, frisée, lamb's lettuce, etc
- 85 g/3 oz taco seasoning mix

Method

Drain the beans and chick peas, combine with green pepper and onion and set aside. Combine all the other ingredients, except the taco seasoning and the mixed leaves. Pour over the bean mix, mixing well. Cover and marinate in the refrigerator overnight or for 24 hours, stirring occasionally.

Drain before serving, leaving a small amount of the marinade. Add the taco seasoning to this, mix and pour over the beans. Serve on a bed of the mixed leaves.

Split Pea and Ham Soup: Serving Size: 6

Another easy recipe that is hard to get wrong!

Ingredients

- 283 g/10 oz split peas
- 1.2 litres/2 pints water
- 1 × 454 g/16 oz tin chicken broth or 1 chicken stock cube made up with 570 ml/1 pint water
- 1 carrot, finely diced
- 2 stalks of celery, sliced
- 1 small onion, chopped
- 170 g/6 oz diced ham (real ham is preferable to prepacked)
- 1 bay leaf
- ½ teaspoon dried tarragon
- Salt and black pepper to taste

Method

Wash the split peas thoroughly. Tip all the ingredients into a casserole and bring to the boil. Reduce heat, and simmer for 2–3 hours, stirring occasionally. Remove the bay leaf and serve.

You can add more flavour by adding a smoked ham hock to the soup while cooking, although EU regulations have made these almost impossible to obtain. For a vegetarian version, omit the ham and use vegetable broth instead of chicken broth.

Bruine Boonen Soupe (Brown Bean Soup): Serving Size: 4–6

Ingredients

- 454 g/16 oz dried brown or frijole negro (black) beans
- 845 ml/1½ pints water
- 170 g/6 oz smoked pork / ham, cubed
- 1 large white onion, diced
- 1 bay leaf
- 4 tablespoons butter
- 2 tablespoons flour
- black pepper

Method

Soak the beans overnight.

Add the pork or ham and the bay leaf, and boil them in the water in which they were soaked; typical cooking time is from 60 to 90 minutes. Skim the soup.

Fry the onion until golden.

Make up the flour and butter into a roux, then add first the onion and then the soup.

Season with black pepper. Salt is not usually needed.

Lentil-stuffed Mushrooms: Serving Size: Approx. 8

Served hot, these stuffed mushroom caps are crispy on top and soft inside.

Ingredients

- 12 to 16 medium mushrooms
- 57 g/2 oz butter or margarine
- 57 g/2 oz onions, finely chopped
- ¼ teaspoon salt
- ⅛ teaspoon freshly ground black pepper

- 113 g/4 oz cup cooked lentils (about 57 g/2 oz dry)
- 113 g/4 oz grated Parmesan cheese (or substitute Cheddar cheese)
- 57 g/2 oz dry wholemeal breadcrumbs

Method

Preheat oven to gas Mark 4/180 °C/ 350 °F.

Remove stems from mushrooms. Chop stems and set aside. Arrange caps in an oiled baking dish.

In a frying pan, stir together butter, chopped stems, onion, salt and pepper. Cook until onions are translucent and soft.

Stir in lentils, cheese and breadcrumbs. Remove from heat.

Stuff caps with the lentil mixture. Bake for 10 to 15 minutes, or grill for about 5 minutes.

Serve hot.

Baked Beans on Toast

A Proustian dish loaded with memories and nutrients. This recipe combines resistant starch with non-digestible fibre ('roughage'), a sprinkling of B vitamins and a smidgeon of lycopene (from the tomato sauce). Don't spoil this by using standard baked beans, which for some unaccountable reason are stuffed with sugar – use a low-sugar version instead and if you have an incurable sweet tooth, add Splenda or aspartame (Canderel) to taste. The toast should of course be wholemeal.

Gourmet tip: a sprinkle of grated cheddar over the top and then 60 seconds under a high grill is good. Poseur tip: use Parmesan.

Ingredients

- Baked beans
- Toast
- Cheese (optional)

Method

You're not serious?

And another easy one. . .

Salmon and Split Pea Paté: Serving Size: 6–8 (3–4 as a main course)

Ingredients

- 1 × 454 g/16 oz tin red salmon
- 227 g/8 oz soft cream cheese (low fat if you're counting every calorie)
- 227 g/8 oz cooked yellow split peas, pureed
- 1 tablespoon lemon juice
- 3 teaspoons grated onion
- 1 teaspoon horseradish or horseradish sauce
- $\frac{1}{4}$ teaspoon salt
- $\frac{1}{4}$ teaspoon Worcester sauce

Method

Drain and clean salmon, blend with remaining ingredients until smooth. Press into a small mould and refrigerate.

Invert mould on to a plate, garnish with parsley or chives, and serve with crackers or crudités.

Lemon Lentil Soup: Serving Size: 4

Excellent with hot wholemeal bread and a green salad.

Ingredients

- 227 g/8 oz green or brown lentils
- 845 ml/1½ pints of vegetable stock, or soup if you must
- 570 ml/1 pint water
- 1 medium onion, finely chopped
- ½ teaspoon oregano

- 113 g/4 oz brown rice
- 1 bay leaf
- ½ teaspoon fresh ground black pepper (or to taste)
- ½ teaspoon pre-packaged curry powder (or to taste)
- 2 lemons

Method

Rinse lentils in strainer until water runs through clear. Put in a large pan (with a lid) along with the brown rice, the vegetable stock and 275 ml/½ pint of water, and bring to the boil. Lower heat to a medium high simmer. Add bay leaf, oregano, pepper and curry powder, cover and cook for 25 minutes.

While the lentils are cooking, saute onion in olive oil until soft (about 5–6 minutes).

When the soup has cooked for 25 minutes, add the sautéed onion. Continue cooking covered for another 20 minutes. Remove bay leaf.

Ladle soup into bowls, and serve each bowl with half a lemon and fresh ground pepper to taste. (Lemon juice is squeezed over the soup according to taste.)

Option: After cooking, the soup can be blended to produce a creamier texture.

Pink Cucumber and Celery Soup: Serving Size: 10

Cool pink, deliciously refreshing and packed with goodness!

Ingredients

- 1 tablespoon unsalted butter
- 3 cucumbers
- 4 large beetroots
- 1 tablespoon olive oil
- 227 g/8 oz flour
- 4 cooking apples, peeled, cored and sliced thin
- 2 medium onions, peeled and chopped
- 227 ml/8 fl oz dry vermouth
- 4 stalks celery, de-stringed and chopped
- 3 pints chicken stock
- 2 cloves garlic, finely chopped
- juice of ¼ lemon
- black pepper and salt (low sodium for preference) to taste
- 170 ml/6 fl oz sour cream
- 227 ml/8 fl oz natural yoghurt

Method

Pre-heat oven to gas Mark 4/180 °C/350 °F.

Peel cucumbers and cut in half lengthways. Use a spoon to scoop out the seeds, and discard them. Grate cucumbers into a colander or sieve, sprinkle with the salt and leave to drain for 30 minutes.

Wash the beets, cut off tops, wrap beets in aluminium foil and bake until tender (1 hour approx.). Allow to cool; peel and dice; set aside.

Combine the butter and olive oil in a large saucepan. Fry the apples, garlic and onions until soft but not brown, add the vermouth and lemon juice and bring to the boil. Add the chopped celery, chopped beets, cucumbers and the chicken stock and allow to cool.

When tepid, pour into a food processor, add the HiMaize and purée. Blend in the sour cream and the yoghurt. Refrigerate and serve cold.

Main Courses

Mexican Stand-off: Serving Size: 4

Ingredients

- 2 tablespoons olive oil
- 1 medium onion, chopped
- 3–5 cloves garlic, minced
- 1 green pepper, finely chopped
- 454 g/1 lb green beans, diced
- 113 g/4 oz Basmati rice (I know this isn't Mexican, but it has a lower GI!!)
- 1 tablespoon chilli powder
- ½ teaspoon salt
- freshly ground black pepper to taste
- 3 tablespoons tomato paste
- 845 ml/1½ pints water
- 1 454 g/16 oz tin kidney beans
- 3 tablespoons parsley, finely chopped
- ½ teaspoon dried oregano

Method

Heat the oil in a large frying pan or wok over a medium-high heat. Add the onion and garlic and saute for about 2 minutes. Stir in the green pepper, green beans, rice, chilli powder, salt and pepper and cook for about 2 minutes, stirring frequently.

Add the tomato paste and the water, and mix well. Allow the contents of the frying pan to come to the boil, cover and simmer for 20–25 minutes until the liquid is absorbed and the rice is cooked.

Remove the pan from the heat, stir in the beans, parsley and oregano. Cover again and allow to stand for 5 minutes.

Serve immediately or allow to cool uncovered, then reheat before serving at a later stage.

Chilli sans Carne: Serving Size: 3–4

Ingredients

- 2 tablespoons olive oil
- 1 onion, chopped
- 1 carrot, chopped
- 3–6 cloves garlic, chopped
- 1 green pepper, chopped
- 1 red pepper, chopped
- 113 g/4 oz green lentils
- ½ teaspoon chilli powder
- 1 teaspoon cumin
- 1 bay leaf
- pinch cayenne pepper
- 1 × 454 g/16 oz tin tomatoes
- 450 ml/¾ pint vegetable stock
- 1 × 454 g/16 oz tin kidney beans, drained
- 1 × 454 g/16 oz tin chick peas, drained

Method

Heat the oil in a pan, add the onion, carrot, garlic and peppers and cook until they are tender.

Add the lentils, spices, tomatoes and the stock. Simmer for 50 minutes.

Add the kidney beans and chick peas, simmer for another 30 to 40 minutes.

Serve with either brown rice, pumpernickel or wholemeal bread. This dish reheats very easily and successfully.

Multi-Bean Stew: Serving Size: 6

This is so easy to make even I can do it!

Ingredients

- 1 red onion, chopped
- 1 tablespoon olive oil
- 2–4 cloves garlic, chopped
- ½ teaspoon paprika (medium hot, or hotter if you can take it)
- 227 g/8 oz cannellini beans
- 227 g/8 oz soy beans
- 227 g/8 oz kidney beans
- 227 g/8 oz green or red lentils
- 1.5 litres/2½ pints water
- 1 bay leaf
- 1 teaspoon celery seed
- 1 teaspoon dill
- 2 teaspoons salt, low sodium for preference
- ¼ teaspoon black pepper, freshly ground is best
- 1 vegetarian stock cube
- 454 g/16 oz diced carrots and/or celery

Method

Sauté the onion and the garlic in oil along with the paprika.

Put all the ingredients in a slow cooker, and simmer on high for about 4 hours or low for 6–8 hours, i.e overnight.

For omnivores, adding ham or bacon is a pretty good idea; just throw 170 g/6 oz of diced ham or smoked bacon into the mix.

Morocco-Bound Chicken and Lentils: Serving Size: 4

Ingredients

- 2 tablespoons olive oil
- 8 chicken drumsticks (1.14 kg/ 2½ lb), skin removed and fat trimmed
- 170 g/6 oz flour
- 227 g/8 oz brown lentils, rinsed
- 6 large spring onions, chopped
- 6 tablespoons chopped coriander
- 85 g/3 oz dried apricots, quartered

- 113 g/4 oz dark raisins
- 57 g/2 oz minced parsley
- 1½ teaspoons grated fresh ginger
- ¼ teaspoon *each* ground allspice, cinnamon, cumin and (cayenne) pepper
- pinch of salt (low-sodium preferred)
- 570 ml/1 pint chicken stock

Method

Heat oven to gas Mark 4/ 180 °C/350 °F. Have ready a large deep ovenproof casserole with a lid.

Heat oil in frying pan over medium heat. Coat chicken with flour, shaking off excess. Fry in batches until browned, about 5 minutes per batch, then set the chicken pieces aside in the casserole.

Drain fat from the frying pan, then add the lentils, spring onions, 4 tablespoons of coriander, apricots, raisins, parsley, ginger, salt and spices. Cook, stirring, for 1 minute.

Empty the contents of the frying pan into the casserole, add the chicken stock and bring to the boil.

Cover the casserole and place in oven. Bake for 30 minutes, uncover and bake for 20 minutes longer or until chicken and lentils are tender. Sprinkle with the remaining coriander.

Black Bean Burritos: Serving Size: 5–6

Ingredients

- 2 × 454 g/16 oz tins of frijole negro (black) beans (or about 227 g/ 8 oz dry)
- 2 carrots, grated
- 2–4 green chillies (depending on your taste buds), plus 1–2 chillies for salsa
- 227 g/8 oz fresh mushrooms, sliced
- 227 g/8 oz tinned tomatoes
- 227 g/8 oz red onion, chopped
- 2–4 cloves garlic
- tortillas, whole wheat if you can find them

Method

If the beans aren't cooked, cook them: rinse thoroughly, add to 570 ml/1 pint of water and simmer for at least 1 hour.

Mix the beans, carrots, chillies and mushrooms in a pan and simmer over a low heat for about 30 minutes.

Meanwhile prepare the salsa: take the tomatoes, the onion, the garlic and 1–2 chillies and either hand chop (arduous), or give them a quick whizz in the food processor so there is still some texture left.

Oil a casserole dish. In each tortilla put a couple of large spoonfuls of the bean, carrot, mushroom and chilli mixture. Fold up the tortillas and place them in the casserole dish, making a layer of tortillas. After each layer, pour on a bit of the sauce from the mixture so that at the end the casserole dish is full of the sauce. Cover, and bake for 40 minutes at gas Mark 4/180 °C/ 350 °F.

Serve with grated cheddar over the top and salsa and guacamole on the side. Sour cream or crème fraîche (half fat for the calorie counters) is pretty good too.

Turkey Red Bean Chilli: Serving Size: 6

Ingredients

- 681 g/1½ lb turkey, chopped finely
- 2 tablespoons olive oil
- 2 onions, diced
- 1 green pepper, diced
- 1 small jalapeno, chopped finely
- 3 cloves garlic, chopped
- ½ tsp chilli powder
- ¼ tsp dried oregano
- ¼ tsp ground cumin
- pinch cinnamon
- 1 × 454 g/16 oz tin tomatoes
- 2 × 454 g/16 oz tins kidney beans
- 1 tablespoon cider or wine vinegar
- 1 tablespoon unsweetened cocoa powder
- salt, to taste

Method

Pour the oil into a casserole, and put over a medium heat. Add the turkey pieces, and cook while stirring until the meat is no longer pink, then for another 5 minutes. Add the onions, pepper, jalapeno and garlic.

Cook for about 4 minutes or until the vegetables are softened. Stir in the chilli powder, oregano, cumin and cinnamon. Cook for 2 minutes.

Stir in the tomatoes and their liquid. Heat to boiling. Reduce heat and simmer, covered, for 25 minutes, stirring once or twice.

Stir in the beans and salt, cover and simmer for 20 minutes.

Stir in the cider vinegar and cocoa powder; stir to combine.

Serve with low fat crème fraîche and a green salad; rocket is good, and fresh tomatoes go well too, as does the occasional pickled gherkin.

Mexican Chicken Pie: Serving Size: 4–6

Ingredients

Pie crust:

- 227 g/8 oz flour
- ¼ teaspoon salt

- 6 tablespoons butter
- 57 ml/2 fl oz ice-cold water

Filling:

- 454 g/1 lb cooked chicken pieces
- 1 medium onion, chopped
- 1 large bell pepper, chopped
- 1 × 454 g/16 oz tin kidney beans, drained
- 284 ml/10 fl oz sour cream or crème fraîche (low fat if you want)

- 2 tbsp Mexican seasoning
- 170 g/6 oz grated cheddar (strong is better)
- 1 teaspoon cayenne (optional – if you like spicy)
- 227 g/8 oz fresh sweet corn or 1 tin sweet corn, drained
- 2 tablespoons olive oil

Method

Pie crust:

Put the flour and salt in the bowl of a food processor. Cut the butter into the flour. Blend for a few seconds until the mix resembles coarse meal. Add the ice-cold water drop by drop, blending all the while – this should take about 30 seconds. Wrap and chill the pastry for 1 hour.

Meanwhile, prepare the filling:

Heat the olive oil in a large pan, add the onion and sauté for 5–8 minutes. Add the pepper and fry for 5 minutes more. Add the corn, kidney beans and seasoning and mix thoroughly over the heat. Set aside, and go back to the pie crust. . .

Lightly flour a flat surface, remove chilled pastry from fridge. Divide pastry in half, pat each half into a flat round. Flour the rolling pin, roll pastry in one direction only, turning it to prevent it sticking to the surface till about 3 mm/⅛ inch thick.

Using the pie dish as a guide, cut out the pastry slightly larger than the pie dish. Fold the pastry in half to make transport easier, and ease it into the pie dish so that it overhangs the edges slightly.

Put the cooked chicken pieces in the pie, pour over the onions, corn, beans, top with sour cream, and sprinkle the grated cheddar over the cream.

Roll out the second piece of pastry, cut as before, fold and drape over the top of the pie. Press top and bottom layers of pastry together, and cut off excess.

Cook in a covered pie dish for 35 minutes at gas Mark 4/ 180 °C/ 350 °F, then uncover and cook for 10 minutes more.

Optional toppings (they're all good):

- Fresh avocado slices or guacamole
- Jalapeno rings
- Simple Salsa

Simple Salsa

In a food processor combine:

- 1 × 454 g/16 oz tin tomatoes with juice
- 1 fresh jalapeno pepper
- 1 green or yellow bell pepper
- 1 medium onion
- ½ large bunch of coriander
- 1–2 fresh tomatoes

Process until fine chopped (but stop before it turns into a slurry). Serve with tortilla chips, if you like.

Spiced Lentils: Serving Size: 6

Ingredients

- 340 g/12 oz dried green lentils
- 2 tablespoons butter
- 2 large cloves of garlic, crushed
- 227 g/8 oz onion, finely chopped
- 1 large stalk celery, chopped
- 454 g/1 lb cooking apple (Bramley or similar) chopped
- 1 teaspoon salt
- 227 g/8 oz shredded coconut
- ½ teaspoon powdered ginger
- ½ teaspoon turmeric
- ½ teaspoon cinnamon
- ½ teaspoon ground coriander
- a few tablespoons of water, as needed
- black pepper, to taste
- juice of one large lemon
- cayenne pepper, to taste

Method

Cook the lentils in 570 ml/1 pint water until tender, topping up the water if needed.

Fry the garlic, onions and celery in butter until tender; then add the apple and cook for a further 10 minutes (covered).

Add the contents of the frying pan to the lentils in a casserole, add the coconut, spices and lemon juice, cover and cook for 45 minutes in the oven at gas Mark 1/140 °C/275 °F.

Omnivorous option: add 227 g/8 oz chicken (small pieces) at the beginning of the frying process.

Baked Stuffed Mackerel with Leek and Lentils: Serving Size: 2

Ingredients

- 2 mackerel, cleaned and fins removed
- 56 g/2 oz feta cheese, cut into small cubes
- 2 teaspoons fresh thyme, chopped
- 4 sundried tomatoes, finely chopped
- lemon juice
- 56 g/2 oz puy lentils
- 1 glass red wine
- 100 ml water
- 1 onion, finely chopped
- 1 large leek, trimmed, cleaned and cut in half, each piece tied around the waist with poultry string
- 275 ml/½ pint vegetable stock

Method

Mix together the cubed feta, sundried tomatoes and fresh thyme with a little olive oil. Then stuff the cavities of the fish. Place the fish in a roasting tray, sprinkle with a little more olive oil and lemon juice and season with black pepper. In a separate pan sweat the onion and garlic gently in a little olive oil until transparent and soft. Add the rinsed puy lentils, pour over the red wine and water and bring up to the simmering point. Let the lentils cook until tender. In a separate pan heat the vegetable stock, drop in the tied-up leeks and allow to poach gently for about 10–15 minutes. When tender, drain and remove the string. Cover the mackerel with tin foil and put in a preheated oven (gas Mark 1/275 °C/140 °F) for about 15 minutes, or until cooked through. Serve the mackerel with the lentils and poached leek.

Wild Salmon Oatcakes with Caper Sauce: Serving Size 2–3 (makes 8 small or 6 large fishcakes)

Salmon Oatcakes

Ingredients

- 1 × 397 g/14 oz tin wild red salmon
- 85 g /3 oz oat flakes
- 57 ml /2 fl oz skimmed milk
- 1 free range egg
- 2 tablespoons dill or chervil, chopped
- salt
- black pepper
- extra virgin olive oil
- 6 tablespoons fresh breadcrumbs

Caper Sauce

Ingredients

- small carton low fat, live natural yoghurt
- 1 pickled gherkin, finely chopped
- 2 tablespoons capers, finely chopped
- salt
- black pepper
- 1 teaspoon chives, chopped

Method

Mix sauce ingredients together, season and chill. Combine together all oatcake ingredients except the olive oil and breadcrumbs. Shape the cakes into rounds about 2 cm/¾ inch thick and roll in the breadcrumbs. Heat a little oil in a non-stick frying pan and brown each fishcake for about 3-4 minutes each side over a medium heat. Serve with the sauce and a wedge of lemon, with Jerusalem artichoke mash and green beans.

Desserts

Pineapple Pushover: Serving Size: 6

This is quite a rich dessert, but when made in this way the glycaemic index is quite low. Still – don't overdo it! As raw eggs are used, the very young, pregnant women and the elderly and infirm should not eat this dish *unless* you are very sure that the eggs used are of a sufficiently high quality.

It can be made the day before.

Ingredients

- 113 g/4 oz Splenda or 3 tablespoons Canderel or 57 g/ 2 oz fruit sugar
- 113 g/4 oz butter
- 2 eggs, beaten
- 2 drops vanilla essence
- 1 × 454 g/16 oz tin pineapple, drained and blended
- 150 ml/¼ pint whipping cream
- 113–170 g/4–6 oz chopped nuts (almonds, brazils, pecans or walnuts are all fine)
- 1 teaspoon fresh grated ginger

Method

Grease a 23 cm/9-inch pan with butter. Sprinkle half the chopped nuts on the bottom of the pan.

Cream the butter and the Splenda, then add the beaten eggs and the vanilla essence. Put this mixture on top of the chopped nuts, layer the pineapple over the top.

Beat the cream stiff. Fold half the remaining nuts into the cream and layer over the pineapple. Sprinkle the remainder of the nuts and the grated ginger over the top, and refrigerate.

Green Jasmine Tea Jelly: Serving Size: 6

Ingredients

- 1 tablespoon gelatine
- 2 tablespoons water
- 845 ml/1½ pints of brewed green jasmine tea, still warm
- sweetener to taste, typically 1 tablespoon Canderel or 1 tablespoon Splenda
- 4 teaspoons lemon juice

Method

In a small bowl, sprinkle the gelatine into the water and allow to stand until softened.

Microwave the gelatine/water mix in 30-second bursts until all the gelatine powder has liquefied, or make up as per directions.

Stir into the tea along with the Canderel, Splenda and lemon juice.

Pour into six small dessert dishes and allow to set in the fridge for at least four hours. Before serving garnish with rose petals, if you have nothing better to do.

You can use green Earl Grey tea if you prefer the bergamot flavour.

Exotic Milk Jelly with Crimson Berry Sauce: Serving Size: 6

Ingredients

Milk Jelly:

- 570 ml/1 pint whole milk
- 1 pack unflavoured gelatine
- 113 g/4 oz Splenda or 3 tablespoons Canderel
- 1 vanilla bean, split
- 6 green cardamom pods, crushed
- zest of 1 lime, grated

Crimson Berry Sauce:

- 454 g/1 lb mixed berries such as raspberries, blueberries, redcurrants, blackberries
- 28 g/1 oz fruit sugar
- 28 g/1 oz Splenda or 1 tablespoon Canderel
- 1 tablespoon fresh lemon juice
- zest of an eighth of a lemon

Method

Milk Jelly:

Place 57 ml/2 fl oz milk in a small bowl, sprinkle over gelatine.

In a saucepan bring the remaining milk, sugar, vanilla, cardamom and lime zest to a boil, stirring to dissolve the Splenda/ Canderel. Remove from the heat, add the softened gelatine and stir well. Cover and leave to infuse for at least 20 minutes.

Meanwhile, rinse the jelly moulds with cold water and set on a flat tray. Strain the milk mixture through a fine sieve. Pour into prepared moulds and refrigerate until set. Turn out on to plates and serve with fresh fruit.

Crimson Berry Sauce:

Blend all the ingredients in a blender (seeds can be strained out if you like).

Pour the berry fruit coulis over the top of the milk jelly – it will look very good against the white jelly shapes. Quite gothic, really.

Indian Fruit Salad: Serving Size: 6

Ingredients

- 2 mangos
- 2 apples
- 1 pear
- 1 papaya
- 227 g/8 oz strawberries
- 227 g/8 oz pineapple, fresh or tinned
- 1 small banana, still slightly green
- 113 g/4 oz black grapes, halved
- 2 tablespoons Splenda or Canderel, or 1 tablespoon fruit sugar
- 2 teaspoons roasted cumin seeds, finely ground
- 2 teaspoons fresh lime juice
- zest of 1 lime
- ½ teaspoon hot paprika

Method

Cut all the fruit in small pieces into a large bowl, and add the lime juice.

Sprinkle the Splenda/Canderel, the spices and the zest over the fruit and mix thoroughly. (This is important, the flavour should be surprising rather than shocking.)

Chocolate Brownies: Serving Size: Up to 12

Normally off the dieter's menu, but even a sinful food can be redeemed by tweaking the recipe. The glycaemic load is lowered by using resistant starch flour, and the dark chocolate adds flavonoids. Although you still shouldn't overdose. . .one or two a day is enough!

Ingredients

- 170 g/6 oz butter
- 340 g/12 oz dark chocolate
- 85 g/3 oz Splenda
- 2 tablespoons instant coffee
- 1 teaspoon vanilla
- ½ teaspoon salt
- 4 large eggs
- 227 g/8 oz flour

Method

Pre-heat oven to gas Mark 4/ 180 °C/375 °F. Butter the pan (I usually use a pie tin).

Melt butter and 142 g/5 oz of chocolate over pan of boiling water. Chop the remaining 198 g/7 oz chocolate coarsely and set aside for later use. Stir the butter and chocolate until smooth.

Remove from heat and add Splenda, coffee, vanilla and salt – then add eggs one at a time.

Toss together the flour and the remaining 198 g/7 oz of chopped chocolate in another bowl and add to the batter. Stir until combined. This is the time to add a handful of nuts if you like them. I prefer walnuts, pecans or tiger nuts.

Bake for 20 minutes.

Resistant Apple Crumble: Serving Size:

Ingredients

- 5 apples, peeled, cored and sliced (cooking apples are best)
- juice from ½ lemon
- 1 teaspoon cinnamon
- 113 g/4 oz Splenda or 85 g/3 oz fruit sugar
- 57 g/2 oz Muscovado brown sugar

- 113 g/4 oz flour
- 227 g/8 oz oats, rolled
- 113 g/4 oz butter (unsalted)
- 113 g/4 oz walnuts (optional)
- 1 teaspoon nutmeg (optional)

Method

Pre-heat oven to gas mark 4/ 180 ° C/350 °F.

Melt butter in a small saucepan over a low heat, when melted stir in the brown sugar. Take off the heat, add flour and oats and mix until all dry ingredients are moist.

Butter a small casserole and press ⅔ of the oat mix across the bottom and sides: set aside.

In a medium bowl combine the apples, lemon juice, cinnamon, nutmeg and the fruit sugar or Splenda. Mix until the apples are coated, place apple pieces in the casserole and crumble the remaining oat mix over them. Now is the time to sprinkle walnut pieces over the top, if you like them.

Cover the casserole and bake for 30 minutes. Remove cover and replace in oven for further 10 minutes to brown.

If feeling sinful, serve with ice cream. If you're not feeling excessively sinful, you could use a low-sugar frozen yoghurt or ice cream.

As an alternative, this pie works really well with a rhubarb or strawberry filling.

CLAYTON PLAN TOP TIP 8

Don't forget the fermentable carbs when dining out. Good restaurant choices include Indian and Moroccan cuisine, both traditionally feature many delicious dishes based on pulses.

8
The Clayton Plan for Exercise

As with diet, there is a plethora of governmental and agency guidelines which purport to tell us how much exercise we should ideally take. We certainly need to take more than we do, because the reality is that most of us today take too little exercise as children, and even these low levels of activity decline as we get older. The typical pattern of changing activity runs down from the football and hockey pitches of our teenage years, via the golf links of middle age to the bowling greens and card tables of old age. This pattern of decline not only mirrors our advancing decrepitude, but also contributes to it, and to our ever-increasing weight.

Where does it all start? At what point did our lifestyles become so very much less physical? Well, quite apart from all the problems associated with life lived in urban or metropolitan spaces, a good deal of this starts in childhood, and with TV. Studies of children's behaviour such as those by Larry Tucker at Brigham Young University in Utah, and Ross Anderson at the Centres for Disease Control, showed that for young children junk TV is just as bad as junk foods. More hours spent watching TV equated with more snacking, less exercise taken and a greater likelihood of overweight and obesity. The almost universal take-up of computer games has increased further the numbers of hours spent in front of screens, and most computer games (with a few honourable exceptions) only exercise the thumb muscles. This is bad enough when the TV or computer game is sited in a communal space; more recent studies have suggested that siting the television or computer in the child's bedroom tends to make matters worse.

It may be an easy option at times to allow the kids to disappear into their room, and into cyberspace. The problem is that obese children are very much more likely to become obese adults, go on to develop any and all of the diseases of overweight, and drive our healthcare system into bankruptcy just at a time when we, the ageing parents, will need it most.

Health Benefits of Exercise

Exercise is not just important for weight control – it also brings immense general health benefits. The facts are startling:

- Studies have shown that inactivity is as great a risk factor for heart disease as a 20-a-day cigarette habit and is as bad as having hypertension or raised cholesterol.[1,2]
- The unfit have two and a half times more risk of early cardiac death than the fit.[3]
- Taking sufficient exercise can override or neutralize bad eating habits.
- Regular exercise lowers blood pressure and improves blood sugar control in diabetics.
- Exercise lowers the level of 'bad' cholesterol and raises the level of 'good' cholesterol.
- Exercise boosts the body's production of its own antioxidant enzymes.

How Much Exercise

We know roughly how much exercise is needed to reduce the risk of illness. Doing 2,500 calories worth of exercise per week reduces the risk of a heart attack, 1 mile of brisk walking per day reduces the risk of developing Type 2 diabetes by up to 58%, and 2,900 calories of exercise per week is sufficient in most cases to maintain a healthy body weight. That may sound like a lot of calories but it is achievable.

Thirty minutes a day of brisk walking gets you into a healthier and leaner condition; an hour a day is even better. For example you could take a half hour walk at lunchtime and, by getting off the bus a stop earlier on the way to and from work, walk 15 minutes in the morning and another 15 minutes in the evening. You will be burning 300 calories per day – that's 2,100 calories each week. Ring the changes by substituting every other day's walk with an hour of heavy gardening, heavy housework (such as high energy hoovering), dancing or jogging, enough in all cases to work up a sweat, and you have already carved out a new lifestyle which will change your body shape and your health prospects.

Testing Your Fitness Level

The easiest way to measure how fit you are is to measure your resting pulse rate. To find your average pulse rate, locate your carotid artery under the jaw or the pulse on your wrist. Using a wrist watch count the number of heart beats for 15 seconds and then multiply by 4 – this gives you your minute reading. Generally, the lower your pulse rate the fitter you are. Check the chart below for a quick assessment.

Resting Pulse Rate

Age	Poor	Fair	Good	Excellent
Men				
20–29	86+	70–84	62–68	60 or less
30–39	86+	72–84	64–70	62 or less
40–49	90+	74–88	66–72	64 or less
50+	90+	76–88	68–74	66 or less
Women				
20–29	96+	78–94	72–76	70 or less
30–39	98+	80–96	72–78	70 or less
40–49	100+	80–98	74–78	72 or less
50+	104+	84–102	76–82	74 or less

For those unable or unwilling to incorporate exercise into the daily routine, the Zenique bath may provide a more acceptable alternative. This system uses muscle stimulation to provide a 10 minute work-out in the bath which preliminary results show to be sufficiently intense to lower blood pressure and blood glucose, if used regularly.[4]

This sort of exercise regime is strongly linked to a reduced risk of Type 2 diabetes, heart disease and colon cancer. In fact, leaner is healthier all over. At the Harvard University School of Public Health, Professors Walter Willett and Meir Stampfer showed that the risk of death increases by 1% for every one pound overweight between the ages of 30 and 49, and by 2% per pound thereafter. In other words, stay lean; getting comfortably fatter as we get older is not natural, and it is not healthy.

But of course there is a lot more that can be done to improve your looks and your health, and much of it requires no effort at all. Some of the more exciting new approaches to issues such as thermogenic food and clothing, which increase the rate at which you burn calories, will be covered in later chapters.

CLAYTON PLAN TOP TIP 9

> **Exercise opportunities can be found in unlikely places. Climb escalators rather than ride them; use the stairs rather than the lift or offer your seat to someone on the bus or train, and stand. Remember, being even a little more active on a daily basis will be more effective than irregular exercise 'bursts'.**

3

FIGHTING DISEASE WITH THE CLAYTON PLAN

- A strong heart and a strong mind
- Preventing diabetes
- Fighting cancer
- Healthy skin and strong bones

9
Vascular Disease, Type 2 Diabetes and the Dementias

Pharmaco-nutrition is a relatively new term, and is quite distinct from classical nutrition. This new method of treatment starts by analysing all the many biochemical and physiological processes which are going wrong in chronic degenerative disease states. Then, rather than focusing on a single problem, as the drug companies do, it puts in place micronutrient regimes designed to rectify as many of the problems as possible. In Appendix 1 I have provided a broad-based micronutrient programme that will bring about health benefits for most people. However, in Chapters 9 and 10, I also explain where additional supplements are necessary for specific diseases. This is not offence, but defence; no magic bullet, but a comprehensive support programme which provides the body's own repair mechanisms with what they need to do their job properly.

The evidence for the effectiveness of nutritional strategies to prevent and fight disease grows stronger every year. Clinical studies are confirming the evidence we already have from healthy diets around the world. Pharmaco-nutrition can be particularly beneficial for diseases that haunt the West, including heart disease, cancer and Type 2 diabetes, diseases in turn often associated with overweight and obesity. In this chapter and the next I explain how adjustments to your diet and a support programme of supplements can help you avoid these diseases.

Heart Disease

Cardiovascular disease – which includes heart attacks and stroke – remains the leading cause of mortality in the developed world. However some countries fare far worse than others. Britain has one of the highest rates of heart disease in the European Union, and the rate is higher than in the United States or Australia. According to a recent World Health Organization report, Irishmen and Scotsmen are three times more likely to die of coronary artery disease than their French counterparts. Their partners are even worse off; women in Belfast or Glasgow are nine times more likely to die of a heart attack than their French sisters.

The fact that Aberdonians are so much more at risk than the citizens of Toulouse is known as the French Paradox. French cuisine, in some areas at least, is at least as rich as Scottish fare. A diet replete with full fat (not to mention unpasteurized) cheese, cream and pâté de fois gras is not really what the doctor ordered – and yet the French, most unfairly, and even despite those appalling French cigarettes, seem to be able to get away with it.

As we touched on earlier, however, a more detailed look at the French statistics reveals a more complex picture. In the north, where the diet is not so very different from the British way of eating, death rates from vascular disease are higher than in the south where the diet is (obviously) Mediterranean. From epidemiological evidence such as this, together with animal studies, cell culture work and a sprinkling of clinical trials, a detailed understanding is emerging of the complex relationships between the food we eat and the diseases we die of, and how these diseases can be stabilized, and forced into reverse.

But to get to this point, we need to re-evaluate the established models of coronary artery disease which have held sway for so long, and which have proved to be such a waste of time and resources.

The Cholesterol Factor

In heart attack sufferers we often see fatty deposits blocking the coronary arteries. The disease process begins with a fatty streak in the lining of the artery, which expands over time until it impedes blood flow in the vessel (causing symptoms such as angina), and then blocks it, causing the heart attack. The fatty material contains cholesterol compounds, which, according to the theory, were derived from excessive levels of cholesterol in the bloodstream, which were in turn derived from excessive amounts of cholesterol in the diet. A diet too high in meat and dairy foods, therefore, would increase the risk of heart attack.

This theory was reinforced by animal models such as the infamous cholesterol-fed rabbits, which also developed atheroma-like lesions in their arteries. The fact that rabbits do not normally eat cholesterol (unless they are the rare carnivorous sort) was ignored. The fact that a diet too high in meat and dairy products was necessarily depleted in fruits and vegetables also went un-noticed. Ministries and departments of health went into overdrive, warning everyone to cut down on cholesterol and fatty foods in general. The pharmaceutical industry followed, rejoicing, and sold vast amounts of cholesterol-lowering drugs.

But the warnings and the drugs were not as helpful as had been predicted. Belatedly, it transpired that at least half of all heart attack victims have normal blood cholesterol levels. In other words, high cholesterol levels are not a good indicator of risk, and by focusing so exclusively on lowering them, doctors and indeed everyone else were overlooking the real question: why was cholesterol migrating into the blood vessel walls?

Inflammation: the Real Problem

We now know that this migration of cholesterol into blood vessel walls is not a primary or causative event, and has relatively little to do with the amount of cholesterol in the diet. It is a secondary event, a consequence of chronic inflammation of the blood vessel walls. In fact, coronary artery disease is now regarded as a chronic inflammatory disease of the arteries, which is called chronic subclinical arteritis or, more commonly, endothelial dysfunction.

Once the inflammatory process is under way, white blood cells migrate from the bloodstream into the sites of inflammation in the vessel walls and die there, depositing cholesterol. As the inflammation develops, the arteries become insensitive to influences that would normally make them dilate. There is normally a balance between the forces that make arteries dilate and those that make them constrict, so when the dilator elements no longer function, the inflamed arteries must constrict. As they do, they drive up the blood pressure. Although the situation is made worse by excessive salt consumption, this is generally not the cause of the problem though it may be a common exacerbating factor.

This explains why hypertension is a risk factor for heart attacks. It is not – as was previously thought – because increased hydraulic stresses on the vessel walls make them more fragile, or drive cholesterol into the tissues, but because both heart attacks and hypertension have a common cause, namely endothelial dysfunction.

But this just pushes the question further back: what causes this chronic inflammation? The answer seems to be that it is caused when the balance between pro- and anti-inflammatory factors is disturbed, so that the inflammatory factors prevail. And these inflammatory factors are many and varied. . .

Inflammatory Factors

The ability to develop inflammatory reactions in the body is absolutely critical, as it is one of our key defences against any agent that could cause disease. It is important that our bodies can mount an adequate inflammatory reaction to destroy bacteria and parasites that could otherwise make us ill. But it is equally important that the inflammation not be allowed to run out of control, to the point where it begins to destroy healthy tissue, because this leads to different forms of disability and disease. Balance, therefore, is all. But that balance is affected by many dietary and other factors.

The inflammatory reaction is increased by, amongst other things:

- a diet high in saturated fats, and low in the omega 3 polyunsaturates found in foods such as salmon, trout and mackerel[1]

- lipid and cholesterol oxidation products (LOPS and COPS). These are generated inside the body if the diet is low in antioxidants, or by oxidative stresses such as smoking or hyperglycaemia, and outside the body by cooking techniques such as frying and/or cooking at high temperatures with animal fats or polyunsaturated oils (mono-unsaturated oils are best for cooking)[2]
- AGE compounds (advanced glycation end products), toxic substances formed when sugar molecules react with other compounds such as proteins. These are formed in foods during high temperature cooking, and also in the body, more so when we eat a diet high in digestible carbohydrates, or become diabetic.[3]

Set against these are the anti-inflammatory factors. These include:

- sterols, compounds found in plant foods such as seeds and grains which are the vegetable equivalent of cholesterol[4]
- the flavonoids, potent anti-inflammatory agents[5] which occur in many fruits, spices and herbs.

The Western Diet – a Heart Disease Nightmare

Seen from this perspective, the modern diet is a recipe for inflammatory diseases such as heart disease. It is high in saturated fats and low in the omega 3 polyunsaturates. It contains low levels of antioxidants, and correspondingly high levels of COPS and LOPS compounds. It is low in the anti-inflammatory sterols and flavonoids. It contains far too much digestible carbohydrate, thus driving up the formation of AGE products inside the body; uses many cooking processes that produce these in our foods; and is low in naturally occurring foods such as the flavonoids that would otherwise slow AGE formation in our bodies. Finally, it is low in the micronutrients required by the processes of tissue healing, which would otherwise repair the damage done by all the above runaway processes.

If, as the years pass, the rate of tissue damage consistently outpaces the rate of healing, our arteries must become more inflamed, more constricted, and more clogged with atheroma. For broadly the same reasons our veins are also inflamed, leading to varicose veins, and our platelets are too sticky, increasing the risk of blood clot formation, heart attacks and strokes.

This is nothing to do with the ageing process. There are cultures where the risk of hypertension and heart disease is low, and does not increase with age. Our Western version of normality, where heart and vascular disease kills one in every two people, is in fact a construct, and nothing more than the consequence of sustained dietary and lifestyle imbalance. So how do we rectify this imbalance, and steer our skewed metabolisms away from disease and towards health?

Ways to a Healthy Heart

To begin with there are the four time-honoured steps to better living as preached by the health authorities:

- give up smoking
- take more exercise
- eat more fruit and vegetables
- lose excess weight.

Such a programme would dramatically improve our health prospects but the statistics tell us, sadly, that these seemingly simple lifestyle changes are hard to implement. We are not smoking noticeably less, we are taking less exercise rather then more, trends in fruit and vegetable consumption are consistently down, and we are heavier than ever.

But there are alternatives. For those who cannot give up tobacco, there are the new clean nicotine delivery systems explained in Chapter 11. And for those who will not or cannot alter their diets, there is pharmaco-nutrition.

The Pharmaco-nutritional Solution

The pharmaco-nutritional approach starts by analysing the many steps of the disease process, and then puts in place a support programme of micro- and phytonutrients designed to rectify every one of the identified metabolic weaknesses.

In the case of vascular disease, this is relatively straightforward. The inflammation in blood vessel walls can be reduced by increasing the intake of the key anti-inflammatory agents, the flavonoids. These important compounds, which are found in foods such as berries and citrus fruits, and in wine and tea, have a set of properties 'designed' to normalize blood vessel function. They are antioxidants and anti-inflammatory agents, and are selectively taken up into the walls of the blood vessels. Once there they switch off inflammation, shutting down the synthesis and release of inflammatory mediators.

The Healthy Heart Diet

The guidelines for healthy heart eating are fairly straightforward and supported by strong clinical evidence reported in a wide range of respected journals:

- Eat plenty of fruit and vegetables, especially the flavonoid-rich foods such as apples, blackberries, walnuts, tomatoes, cabbage and lettuce.
- Drink a large glass (350 ml/0.75 pint) of citrus juice everyday.
- Eat plenty of vitamin K in the form of spinach, kale or broccoli.
- Cut back on margarines and polyunsaturated vegetable oils; switch to mono-unsaturates such as olive or rape-seed oil.
- Most types of bean and oat-based foods can help reduce blood cholesterol levels, so increase foods such as lentils, frijole negro (black) beans, chick peas, red kidney beans and porridge in your diet.
- Eat oily fish such as trout, salmon or mackerel twice a week.

They also block the effects of enzymes in the walls of the arteries that cause constriction, and stimulate the synthesis of compounds that make the arteries dilate.

Accordingly, the short-term result of flavonoid therapy is the well-documented restoration of the arteries' ability to respond to vasodilators such as acetylcholine.[6] A gradual lowering (normalization) of blood pressure follows, as the inflammation in the walls of the arteries calms down, enabling the vessels to relax and open up and, in the longer term, there is a stabilization of atheroma formation. At the same time, the flavonoids are making the blood platelets less sticky and less reactive, thus reducing the risk of blood clots.

This cloud of vaso- and cardio-protective effects is so considerable and so coordinated that you would imagine that the flavonoids must be vitamins – and in fact their discoverer, the great Hungarian biochemist Albert Szent-Gyorgyi who won a Nobel Prize in 1937 for his work on vitamin C, originally identified the flavonoids as vitamin P.

Following Szent-Gyorgyi's discovery the pharmaceutical companies brought out a range of medicines containing vitamin P, but by the 1960s most had disappeared. Vitamin P could not be patented, and because nobody knew what P was, how best to measure it or even whether it was a single compound or a group of related compounds, the drug industry found it almost impossible to produce standardized and reliable products.

Incidentally, the statins – a class of drug which are now being sold almost like sweets over the counter in some pharmacies – and which were originally thought to protect against heart attacks by reducing cholesterol, have now been found to act as anti-inflammatory agents. In this respect they are just like flavonoids, but far more expensive and very much more prone to causing toxic reactions.[7]

You would be unwise, however, to rely exclusively on either flavonoids or statins for protection. This is because if you live a Western lifestyle, your arteries may well be inflamed – but many other elements in your metabolism are also awry.

Metabolic Problems

For example, a diet which contains high levels of protein and low levels of methyl groups (which are provided by vitamin B6, folic acid, choline and betaine – a nutrient found in sugar beet, sugar cane, prawns, shrimps and eggs), drives up levels of homocysteine in the blood. Excess levels of homocysteine are linked to an increased risk of heart attack and stroke, possibly because this may exacerbate endothelial dysfunction.[8] Taking B vitamins to lower plasma homocysteine levels is not enough on its own to reduce the risk of heart problems – but is a very logical additional ingredient in the flavonoid-based programme.

A more heavily weighted risk factor than homocysteine glyco-sylated haemoglobin (HbAlc for short). In simple terms, this means that molecules in red blood cells have become chemically linked to glucose. While HbA1c is not itself dangerous, the extent to which haemoglobin is glycosylated reflects long-term levels of glucose in the bloodstream, which is in turn a measure of how well blood glucose is controlled. A diet with too high a gly-caemic load (GL) (too reliant on digestible carbohydrates), com-bined with an inactive lifestyle, generally leads to glucose intolerance and Type 2 diabetes, excessive levels of glucose in the blood, and excessive rates of protein glycosylation, where glucose molecules react with and stick to proteins.

When this happens to a protein, its structure changes, gener-ally leading to a loss of that protein's function. If the protein thus affected is in the lens of the eye, the crystalline structure of the lens is disrupted and the lens becomes opaque, forming a cataract. If the protein is in the filtration units in the kidney, the ability of the kidney to filter urine is impaired, a factor contrib-uting to renal disease. And if the protein is in the walls of an artery it becomes less elastic, the artery becomes less able to dilate, and blood pressure starts to increase.

Logically, therefore, a diet with a lower GL is indicated, together with physical exercise. But to this we can add, again, the flavonoids, which have an additional trick up their sleeve, namely their ability to inhibit glycosylation reactions.

Daily Healthy Heart Supplement Regime

A daily supplement regime to reduce heart disease risk should include:

• Vitamin E (mixed tocopherols)	60–70 mg
• Vitamin C	500 mg
• Folic acid	200 mcg
• Calcium	100 mg
• Magnesium	50 mg
• Mixed carotenoids	5–25 mg
• Flavonoid complex	500–1500 mg
• Q10	30–60 mg
• B vitamins	300% of RDA
• Copper as chelate	2 mg
• Zinc as chelate	10 mg
• Selenium	150 mcg
• Betaine	450 mg
• Vitamin K	100 mcg

To this regime add the classic antioxidants, such as vitamins C and E and the mineral selenium. They are ineffective on their own, but are an invaluable addition to the pharmaco-nutritional regime if you wish to reduce the risk of vascular disease still further. To this very substantial support programme you can legitimately add the other antioxidant co-factors copper, zinc and manganese, with iron generally only useful in women of child-bearing age, and a little fish oil.

If the blood pressure remains high, salt substitutes such as PanSalt have been shown to be as effective as anti-hypertensive medication – with the advantage that PanSalt is cheaper and does not cause side-effects. In Finland, where PanSalt was introduced into a wide range of processed foods in the early 1990s, the national average diastolic blood pressure fell within two years by around 8 mm of mercury.[9] This is the equivalent of putting every man, woman and child on anti-hypertensive drugs, and contributed to the over 50% reduction in heart attacks and strokes which occurred at that time. PanSalt is not used in British foods because it would add as much as 1p to the price of a loaf of bread. (It is sold in the US as Cardia.)[10]

When you understand how many links there are in the complex sequence of events that starts with a fatty streak in the artery wall and ends with a heart attack or stroke, the clinical trials that attempted to reduce the risk of heart attacks with limited and arbitrary combinations of micronutrients (such as vitamins C and E) appear simplistic and misguided. Those trials represent the pharmaceutical approach to disease, and are based on a 'magic bullet' model which is narrowly focused on single enzymes, receptors or hormones. In contrast, the pharmaco-nutritional strategy provides a comprehensive support programme, designed to undo the harm caused by our contemporary lifestyles and to provide the elements that our innate healing mechanisms need in order to do their job properly.

Type 2 Diabetes

The same approach can be used in Type 2 diabetes, which is increasingly regarded by clinicians as an accelerated form of cardiovascular disease, or even an accelerated form of ageing.

People with diabetes are particularly prone to vascular problems associated with heart disease, including heart attacks and stroke; impotence; loss of sight due to retinal bleeding and cataract; kidney damage; peripheral neural damage and various other disorders. It is no coincidence that diabetics are also particularly exposed to oxidative stress and excessive glycosylation, two of the mechanisms that drive the ageing process. From this perspective we can see that diabetics need much the same sort of pharmaco-nutritional support as do heart attack candidates, except that, as their metabolic stresses are greater, they require rather higher doses of some of the antioxidants and anti-glycosylants.

Together with a programme of weight loss, exercise and a low GL diet (i.e. less starch and sugars, more fermentable carbohydrates), the condition of most diabetics should be improved if not normalized.

'Experiments' like this have been done in parts of Australia where Aborigines, when exposed to the Western diet, develop frighteningly high rates of Type 2 diabetes and heart disease. In one case the local doctor became so concerned that he decided to encourage the Aborigines to leave the township and resume their traditional lifestyle. It is reported that within a few months their blood pressure, cholesterol and glucose had returned to normal; reverting to their traditional diet of bush food (high in flavonoids, protein and fermentable carbohydrates, and low in digestible carbohydrates), together with increased levels of physical exercise, had effectively cured them.[11]

Super-Sizing

This devastating comment on the dangers of the Western diet, particularly junk foods, was supported recently by the exploits of Morgan Spurlock. Morgan was a healthy 33-year-old American who documented the effects on his body of eating three meals a day at McDonald's, many of which were super-sized, for 30 days. He gained 11 kg (25 lb) in weight, his cholesterol shot up from 165 to 230, his blood glucose responses deteriorated and his liver enzyme results became so abnormal that his doctors urged him to quit – as shown in the film *Super Size Me*.

'Morgan was an extremely healthy person who got very sick eating this McDonald's diet,' his GP Dr Isaacs told the *New York Post*. 'None of us imagined he could deteriorate this badly – he

Digestible Carbs – the Chief Culprits

Remember digestible carbs are those made from refined flour and often with a high sugar content. The main suspects are:

- white bread, rolls, croissants
- commercially made biscuits, cakes and pastries
- potatoes
- confectionery
- soft drinks sweetened with sugar.

looked terrible. The liver test was the most shocking thing – it became very, very abnormal.'

Morgan's diet was admittedly exceptional. In a press release issued by McDonald's, the company states that Morgan was acting irresponsibly by consuming more than 5,000 calories a day and by limiting his physical activity.[12] Nevertheless, this provides an illustration of the close relationship between diet and health; a relationship demonstrated by the staggering increases in diabetes occurring in every developed nation today. The lesson is simple: if your diet is making you sick, don't reach for the pill bottle, which will only suppress the symptoms of your disease. Change your diet and lifestyle, and cure yourself.

Controlling Blood Glucose Levels

There are three basic elements that determine blood glucose levels, and how well they are controlled:

- The amount of digestible carbohydrate you eat. Most of us eat a diet containing far too much digestible carbohydrate. It pours about ten times more glucose into our bloodstreams than we were designed to cope with.
- The size and functionality of our muscles, the glucose 'sinks' into which blood glucose can be cleared. Our high technology society makes us so inactive that our skeletal muscle is too poorly developed to perform its metabolic function of acting as a glucose sink.
- The efficiency with which the hormone insulin stimulates the uptake of glucose into those sinks. The prevalence of Type B malnutrition means that many of us are depleted in the co-factors needed for the glucose uptake pumps to work properly. These require chromium, manganese and, according to recent studies, vitamin D; depletion in any or all of these micronutrients leaves the uptake pumps impaired.

Thanks to our modern times, all three components are fundamentally out of kilter.

To make matters worse, as blood glucose control begins to slip, many proteins in the blood and on cell membranes become glycosylated. Once insulin is glycosylated, its shape changes and it is no longer capable of activating the glucose uptake pumps. It is probable that the insulin receptor also becomes glycosylated and, in this condition, no longer recognizes insulin. These two factors, together with the depletion in chromium and manganese, lead to 'insulin resistance' whereby ever-higher levels of insulin in the blood are needed to control blood sugar levels.

The Solution

The solution, like the problem, is three-fold.

- Reduce the amount of digestible carbohydrate in the diet, replacing it with alternatives such as fermentable carbohydrate.
- Increase exercise levels, which can be combined with or alternated with controlled cold exposure (see Chapter 14).

The Anti-Diabetic Diet

The positive effects of changes in diet to prevent Type 2 diabetes are well documented.

- It's important to switch to foods with a low glycaemic index, such as oat-based foods (e.g. porridge, oat cereals), whole grain foods, pulses, legumes and wholemeal pasta.
- Choose antioxidant-rich foods, particularly foods high in Vitamin E – such as sunflower seeds, sesame seeds and wheatgerm – and in Vitamin C.
- Eat more oily fish and nuts.
- Try to increase your intake of flavonoids, such as grapeseed extract or turmeric.
- Eat fewer meat and dairy products, more vegetable protein-based foods.

- Use a pharmaco-nutritional programme which provides chromium and manganese[13] to support the glucose uptake pumps and flavonoids, which protect against glycosylation and so shield both insulin and the insulin receptors. (If manganese is to be supplemented, it is advisable to co-supplement with copper and zinc also.) Interestingly, given the developing awareness of an inflammatory component in diabetes, the flavonoids' potent anti-inflammatory effects are very likely to play a role here too.

Before moving on to discuss the dementias (which are often linked to the vascular diseases), we must complete our review of diabetes by referring to some of the other specific problems that people with diabetes are likely to encounter. These include bladder and kidney infection, retinal bleeding, and damage to the peripheral nerves which can lead to gangrene and impotence.

Other Diabetic Problems

The problems of bladder and kidney infection are caused by a number of factors, which include a degree of impairment of the immune system, incomplete bladder emptying due to nerve damage, and a probable increase in the numbers of bacterial docking sites in the urinary tract as a consequence of glycolysis. All of these are partially or largely reversible.

Provided that blood sugar can be brought under control, the degree of glycosylation of the tissues can be reduced, and the numbers of bacterial docking sites cut back to normal. A Type B replenishment micronutrient support programme such as the one described for heart disease should help to enhance immune function. If the nerve damage is not too long-standing, it may be possible to achieve some restoration of the nerve cell membranes and function with a combination of the appropriate antioxidants, and phospholipids in foods such as lecithin (in egg yolks and offal). This type of programme should also help to reduce the risk of damage to the peripheral nerves.

If urinary tract infections are still occurring, there is cranberry juice, shown in two studies to reduce the severity and frequency of these infections.[14] The flavonoids in cranberry juice work by dislodging urinary tract bacteria from their docking points, so that they can be flushed out in the urine. If you don't like cranberry juice, the sugar mannose can be used to achieve the same effect. (Mannose is considered too novel to be approved as a food supplement in the European Union, but can be bought freely in the US and over the web.[15])

The problems of loss of sight which affect people with diabetes are caused by cataract and retinal micro-angiopathy, a condition where the tiny blood vessels that supply the retina develop micro-bleeds and proliferate over the surface of the retina. Improved blood glucose control reduces the risk of both of these conditions, but the flavonoids, with their anti-inflammatory and capillary-stabilizing actions, are ideally suited to provide additional protection. Several studies have indicated that they do indeed protect the diabetic retina, so here is another reason for people with diabetes to include high dose flavonoids in their dietary regime.[16] Flavonoids may offer some protection against cataract also, but the evidence here is less clear-cut and suggests that it would make better sense to combine them with wide-spectrum antioxidants.

Dementia

The reason why dementia is bracketed together with vascular disease and diabetes is that many of the same disease mechanisms are involved in all three conditions. For example, the two main causes of dementia are multiple infarcts ('mini-strokes'), and Alzheimer's disease, which may occur separately or together in different patients, and in both these conditions vascular health and oxidative stress play an important role.

Strokes occur when the blood supply to an area of the brain is disrupted, so that the tissue supplied by that artery dies. Stoppages affecting the blood supply to the brain can be caused by either the rupture of a blood vessel ('haemorrhagic stroke'), or by a blockage in a blood vessel ('thrombo-embolic stroke'). Haemorrhagic stroke is generally due to hypertension, which is largely caused by inflammation of the blood vessels, and is therefore logically prevented by the same pharmaco-nutritional programmes used to protect against coronary artery disease. Thrombo-embolic stroke is generally a sequel to disturbances in clotting mechanisms; these too are largely caused by the same factors that predispose to inflamed blood vessels, and will be prevented by the same programme. In both cases stopping smoking, exercise regimes, and controlling weight and blood glucose are important.

Alzheimer's Disease

In Alzheimer's disease, the mechanisms that drive the condition are rather different. Here, there is a progressive loss of certain sub-types of brain cell, specifically those nerves that utilize the neurotransmitter acetylcholine. The pharmaceutical response has been to use drugs such as Aricept which slow or prevent the breakdown of acetylcholine, thereby amplifying its effect. This is not a curative treatment, but merely enhances the effects of the dying population of brain cells, in a way that was thought to improve the patient's overall abilities.

There are 39,000 patients in the UK on these drugs, and at around £1,000 per year per patient the cost of these drugs to the nation is £39 million per year. A recent independently funded study[17] shows that their effect is almost negligible, and achieved at a cost far in excess of more effective and simpler measures such as improved nursing. Yet we continue to use these drugs because we want to do something, and because the pharmaceutical model tells us that this is the logical treatment for Alzheimer's. But the model is wrong.

The real question is not why levels of acetylcholine in the brain fall, but why the cholinergic neurons are dying. This has little to do with the way in which the neurotransmitter is formed or broken down, and is probably everything to do with the dynamics of the nerve cell membranes. But as the elements that affect the cell membranes are micronutrients that cannot be patented and hence cannot be developed into drugs, this area has remained scandalously underdeveloped.

It's not as if there aren't enough clues. Many studies have shown that the risk of developing Alzheimer's is reduced in populations with higher intakes of various micronutrients, including the antioxidant vitamins and minerals, the B vitamins, and other dietary compounds such as the flavonoids (again!).[18] Other researchers working with animal models have shown that the age-related loss of brain cells can be prevented altogether when the diet is augmented with plant and herb extracts containing many of the same phytonutrients, or with the micronutrients alpha-lipoic acid and acetylcarnitine (whose richest source is red meat).[19]

Researchers have also shown that in Alzheimer's, the lesions that occur in the brain – the so-called plaques and tangles – create free radicals that destroy elements in nerve cell membranes.[20] Taken together, these pieces of information create a composite and very persuasive picture, and one which holds out real hope for all of us who worry about this erosive condition.

Prevention and Recovery

The membranes of all our body's cells are dynamic, and are constantly turning over. Structural molecules in the membranes are continually being broken down, and continually being replaced by new ones. If the rate of breakdown and loss is balanced by the rate of replacement, no harm ensues. The cell membranes remain functional, and the cells remain viable. On a poor diet, however, the rate of loss increases and the rate of repair falls. This eventually leads to increasing disrepair of the membrane, poor functioning of nerves, membrane breakdown and the death of the cell.

The membranes of nerve cells contain, as do all cell membranes, molecules called phospholipids. These molecules in turn contain fatty acids, a high proportion of which are polyunsaturated. Polyunsaturated fatty acids are very vulnerable to oxidative stress; lipids account for 60% of the brain's dry weight, and the bulk of these are polyunsaturates. To make matters worse, there is a lot of oxygen in brain tissue; the brain takes up to a quarter of the cardiac output of oxygenated blood, even though it is only 3% of the body's weight. Even worse, the brain's antioxidant defences are not thought to be very high, and as a final touch, some breakdown compounds formed in the brain are actively pro-oxidant.

This is a recipe for cumulative oxidative damage which would inevitably lead to loss of structural units in the nerve cell membranes, loss of cell membrane integrity, and eventual cell death. This would explain why diets high in antioxidants are protective – but it explains some other findings too.

A Brain Protective Diet

When phospholipids have been destroyed by oxidative stress or though some other mechanism, they must be replaced if the cell membrane is not to fail. The replacement phospholipids come from two sources; they are either derived from the diet, or must be manufactured in the liver. Unfortunately, levels of phospholipids in the diet have fallen markedly in the last century, as the main sources of these compounds – crude, cold-pressed vegetable oils and offal meats – have largely disappeared from the food chain. Eggs, the other main source, have been stigmatized as sources of salmonella and cholesterol, and as a result egg consumption fell throughout the 1990s. It was only in 2000 that the egg industry started to try to compensate for this with programs of disease eradication and health promotion.

Under normal circumstances, it is possible to compensate for a dietary lack of phospholipids by manufacturing them in the liver, from simple precursors (molecules from which another molecule or tissue is found) such as glycerol and the fatty acids. This is quite a complex synthesis which requires at least five co-factors (micronutrients and methyl groups), together with an adequate supply of the different types of fatty acids including the omega 3 polyunsaturates. The modern diet tends to be depleted in all of these, and as a result the ability of the liver to produce phospholipids is often less than satisfactory. This is demonstrated by the high numbers of people with fatty livers (where fats accumulate because they cannot be made into the more soluble phospholipids) and/or low levels of HDL cholesterol, which consists largely of liver-derived phospholipids.

Essential Oils

There are two families of essential polyunsaturated fatty acids, omega 6 and omega 3. Like vitamins, these oils are essential for the healthy functioning of every cell in our body, but our body can't produce them – they must be gained from what we eat. Omega 6 is found in many vegetable oils, and at high levels in evening primrose oil, borage and blackcurrant seed oil. Omega 3 is found in oily fish such as salmon, trout, herring and mackerel.

Perhaps now we can begin to understand why Alzheimer's is a disease of old age. There is considerable evidence that as we age, the degree and extent of Type B malnutrition tends to worsen. Poverty, loss of teeth, appetite and the sense of taste, and difficulties in swallowing conspire so that with every passing decade our diets and intakes of the many vital micro- and phytonutrients become progressively compromised.

We become progressively more depleted both in the factors needed to slow the breakdown of phospholipids (broadly, the antioxidants), and the co-factors needed to make new ones. This imbalance leads to a progressive loss of critical structural elements in the nerve cell membranes, which become dysfunctional and then begin to die. Nerves which use acetylcholine have specific requirements and properties that make them especially vulnerable – which is probably why these nerve cells die first.

Genetic risk factors for Alzheimer's are also known, of course, as they are for every disease; but the fundamental truth – and one acknowledged by increasing numbers of neuroscientists – is that the vast majority of us do not have to lose brain cells as we get older, *if* we provide the nutrients that the brain needs to maintain itself.

But it is not all a matter of nutrition. There is evidence that depressive illness is a risk factor for Alzheimer's. This is thought to be because, during depression, the stress hormone cortisol increases in the blood to levels which damage nerve cells and the brain itself – a process which tends to worsen with age.

Chronic stress boosts levels of cortisol in a very similar way, which is why when you are very stressed you become more forgetful. Learning a stress-reduction technique, therefore, may be equally important in maintaining a full count of brain cells.

Cooking your own food, from fresh ingredients, provides a way of improving your micronutrient intake and de-stressing at the same time. Sadly, eating at home seems to be going out of style. As more of us eat out, increasing numbers of houses are being built in the US and latterly in Britain without kitchens, with just space for a freezer and a microwave. But do we really want more fast food? Perhaps what we really need is slow food. . .

For those interested in the slow food concept of sustainable and ethical food production, and the joys of food preparation and, of course, eating, visit www.slowfood.com.

CLAYTON PLAN TOP TIP 10

Wild Salmon Oatcakes (see Chapter 7) are packed with cardio-protective ingredients. Salmon is rich in omega 3 oils, oats can lower total blood cholesterol and eggs increase the level of 'good' HDL cholesterol. They're great for dinner, or eat them cold for lunch the next day.

10
Joints, Bones, Skin and Cancer: The Regeneration Game

In this chapter I want to introduce you to a new way of thinking about the body. Forget the old classifications into bodily systems such as cardiovascular, musculoskeletal, respiratory and the rest. This new way of looking at the body may be less familiar, but it offers critical new insights into the processes of tissue breakdown and healing, and allows us not only to accelerate the healing process, but in certain cases to reverse the effects of the ageing process.

The Matrix

In this new approach we think of the body as being made up of just three components: cells, extra-cellular fluids such as blood, and the extra-cellular matrix. Cells are basically soft, wet and fragile – and the reason we are not is the extra-cellular matrix. This is an ultra-fine three-dimensional mesh of microfibres that holds all our cells in place. If you could wave a wand at someone you don't like – a current political figure, for example – and wish all their cells away, what would remain would be the figure of the person, identical in every way but constructed of an intricate and empty mesh of gauze-like microfibres.

There are basically two types of microfibre, each of which consists of chains of single units strung together. One type is built up from amino acids into fibrous proteins such as collagen and elastin. The other is built up from amino sugars such as glutamine into complex fibre polymers called glycosaminoglycans and proteoglycans. These basic fibres make up the extra-cellular matrix – but the nature of the matrix differs subtly in different parts of the body. The ratio of the different fibre types changes in different regions, depending on the nature, function and workload of the tissue in that region.

You could look at the matrix as an ultra-skeleton. It holds all the cells in any one area or organ together and in the correct alignment, determining the stretchiness, slipperiness, tensile strength or elasticity of each bit of tissue. It provides firmness to the skin, and determines its capacity to hold moisture; it gives elasticity to the arteries, tensile strength to the ligaments, slipperiness and compressibility to the cartilage plates in your joints, and resilience to your bones, which, without the very slight degree of flexibility provided by the matrix microfibres, would shatter every time you barked your shins.

The matrix is constantly being broken down and, in health, as constantly repaired. This shows up as rapid healing of cuts or broken bones, or in the maintenance of healthy joints. Problems can arise, however, when the rate of breakdown exceeds the rate of repair. This can happen when breakdown accelerates, as in inflammation, or when repair slows, as it does in old age or in Type B malnutrition. When the rate of breakdown predominates, skin wrinkles and becomes less elastic; cartilage plates thin and joints become painful; bone starts to erode and muscles to atrophy.

If that sounds like a description of the ageing process, it's no surprise. As we get older, deteriorating dietary habits leave us with progressively worsening Type B malnutrition. We become increasingly depleted in the micronutrients needed for growth and repair, and the micro- and phytonutrients needed to slow the processes of decay and breakdown. Repair and regeneration slow, breakdown accelerates, our tissues gradually become less functional and more prone to cause the symptoms of malfunction that we call disease, all part of the inevitability of ageing.

Except that it is clearly not inevitable. In the last two decades we have learned that this aspect of the ageing process can be reversed. By providing in the diet the nutritional compounds that the processes of healing and repair need, the balance between repair and breakdown can be shifted, so that repair and renewal are once again dominant.

Joints

The best example of this is in osteoarthritis. Joints – are a particularly specialized part of the matrix consisting almost exclusively of fibres made up of glucosamine units – wear thin as we age, and at a certain point, after 20 or 30 years of slow erosion, they become painful. At this late stage in the process of decline, the doctor diagnoses osteoarthritis and prescribes an anti-inflammatory analgesic. These drugs suppress the symptom of inflammation, but do nothing to change the ongoing process of decline, which continues. They do, however, cause a high incidence of side-effects, and are responsible for many hospitalizations due to such problems as peptic ulceration, kidney damage and blood disorders.

Glucosamine – the Joint Repairer

Then glucosamine arrived on the scene. Discovered originally by surgeons who used it to speed wound healing after surgery, glucosamine has been shown in many studies to improve symptoms in arthritic patients, not within hours, as the drugs do, but after a month or two of continuous use.[1]

Why is the onset of action so slow? Because glucosamine is not an anti-inflammatory agent, but an agent of renewal. Cells that lie at the base of the cartilage plates, called chondroblasts, take up glucosamine and build it into microfibres that form the bulk of cartilage itself. Normally chondroblasts make their own glucosamine by combining glucose with the amino acid glutamine. With age, however, the rate of glucosamine synthesis slows, and this slows down the formation of cartilage. By supplying glucosamine in supplement form the initial rate-limiting step is bypassed and the rate of cartilage regeneration speeds up dramatically until it exceeds the rate of cartilage breakdown.

Now, little by little, the cartilage plate starts to grow, until after a few months it has regained enough of its thickness and strength to function properly once more. The joint has effectively been renewed, a relatively slow but genuinely curative approach to osteoarthritis which is far more profound than the fast-acting but merely symptomatic anti-arthritis drugs. I can vouch for this, having seen, in Norway, serial arthroscopic images which clearly show the regeneration of old and worn-out joints in patients who had formerly been crippled by their disease.

Optimum Intake of Glucosamine

To prevent the onset of osteoarthritis, look for a glucosamine supplement of 500 mg per day. To treat an existing condition take 1–2 g daily and combine with 100 mcg vitamin K, 2 mg manganese, 500 mg betaine and 500 to 1500 mg curcumin. Glucosamine hydrochloride is probably the best form.

You can imagine that the pharmaceutical industry, which makes a good deal of money selling their anti-inflammatory drugs, would be concerned by this – and indeed they are. In Sweden, the drugs industry was so concerned by increasing sales of glucosamine supplements that they lobbied the state regulatory agency, who promptly obliged by saying that as glucosamine was so effective, it must be a medicine.[2] This meant that glucosamine could no longer be bought and sold as a supplement, but could only be purchased as a (much more expensive) drug, supplied, naturally, by a pharmaceutical company.

Healthy Teeth

Another example of the dynamism of living tissue is found in the teeth. This might come as a surprise, as the teeth are so stable that they are often the only fossil remains that survive the long passage of time. But dynamism is the only way to understand the concept of re-mineralization, a process in which the enamel of a tooth can heal itself, and put into reverse the early signs of decay. It works like this. . .

Dental enamel is a crystalline material consisting mainly of a calcium phosphate mineral complex called hydroxyapatite. As the teeth are constantly bathed in saliva, there is a constant exchange between mineral ions in the enamel, and in the saliva. If a sugar-free diet is eaten the exchange is on a relatively small scale, and the numbers of ions lost are equalled by the numbers of ions replaced. The enamel retains its density and strength, and there is little if any dental decay.

On a high-sugar Western diet, however, oral bacteria break the ingested sugars down into acids. These dramatically increase the rate at which mineral ions leave the enamel, so that the rate of loss now far outstrips the rate of replacement. There is a net loss of minerals, day by day, so that the enamel becomes etched and eroded and, as demineralization continues, the process of dental decay gets under way.

Take sugar out of the diet, or chew xylitol chewing gum, and the bacteria in the mouth can no longer produce acids. If you're using xylitol gum, the xylitol selectively kills off the bacteria responsible for forming acid, and at the same time forms complexes with the minerals and enhances uptake back into the enamel. Now the rate of mineral replacement outstrips the rate of mineral loss, and re-mineralization occurs. After a while, incipient decay in the teeth begins to resolve, and the enamel re-forms where it was.

The first trials of xylitol gum were carried out in Finland by Professor Makinen at the University of Turku. The results were so unambiguous that the use of xylitol chewing gum is now encouraged throughout the school system, and you can go from classroom to classroom and be treated to the sight of an entire school's worth of children opening their mouths to reveal no fillings.

Public education has done a great deal to make this situation possible in Finland; unfortunately we in the UK are unable to find out much about this sort of thing because the European

Union forbids gum manufacturers from stating on the pack that xylitol gum prevents tooth decay. That would be a medical claim, and making such claims about food is expressly prohibited.

A Micronutrient Support Programme

But back, for the moment, to the joints. . . We discussed glucosamine, but there is more to building a joint than glucosamine. When the chondroblasts build glucosamine into the larger molecules that make up cartilage, they also need the trace element manganese. And as the joint is rather more complex than just cartilage, other micronutrients such as vitamin C, copper, the B vitamins, methyl groups and a number of others should all be wrapped up into a joint support programme. Collagen hydrolysate has a role to play also, as do certain phospholipids which contribute to the lubrication within the joint.

If you have Type B malnutrition, you will be depleted in all of these, and depleted also in the anti-inflammatory agents such as the flavonoids which normally retard rates of joint wear. A broad-spectrum micronutrient support programme should, therefore, push you into renewal mode and restore the joint. It should then maintain the processes of joint wear and replacement in perfect balance – just as they were when you were younger and healthier.

Critically, adequate healing can only be achieved if the disease process is treated at an early stage. If the arthritis has been left untreated or merely treated with palliative anti-inflammatory drugs, it may well have reached a state where the cartilage plate has been effectively destroyed. If there are no chondroblasts left to start up the process of healing, micronutrient support programmes can have no effect.

Rheumatoid Arthritis

Rheumatoid arthritis is another situation entirely. Here, glucosamine is not only ineffective but contra-indicated. In rheumatoid arthritis, the process of inflammation and hence the rate of cartilage loss is so great that glucosamine supplements cannot boost the rates of tissue repair sufficiently to keep up. In the past some patients with rheumatoid arthritis attempted to self-medicate with glucosamine, and as a result did not go to their doctors until the disease had progressed to a point where even the most powerful (and toxic) drugs were of little use.

There is an alternative course of action, however that patients with rheumatoid arthritis might care to explore. In phase 1, the inflammation is brought under control using a combination of sterols (which are immuno-modulatory agents, see page 67), and flavonoids, such as ginger or turmeric, which exert powerful anti-inflammatory effects. Once the inflammation has been damped down, a joint regeneration programme can be implemented with glucosamine, manganese and all the ancillary micronutrients, such as vitamin C, the B vitamins, copper and zinc.

Bones

Moving on from cartilage to bones is a relatively small step; bone, like cartilage, can be regarded as a specialized form of the all-pervasive extra-cellular matrix. It contains most of the same types of microfibre, but in different proportions, as it has very different engineering requirements. Where cartilage must be compressible and slippery, bone must be relatively rigid and yet not brittle. To achieve this the fibre mix contains far more proteins, and the matrix itself becomes mineralized.

As in the joints and teeth, the dynamism displayed by all living tissue plays a central role in determining the health and integrity of the skeleton. Bone turns over very slowly, and you grow a new skeleton every ten years or so. The process is imperceptible, of course, and highly efficient, except that as we age the rate of erosion speeds up and the rate of regeneration slows down. There is a slow net loss of bone, and eventually too many of us develop the brittle bone disease, osteoporosis.

Osteoporosis

How can we reverse this process? A broad-spectrum micronutrient programme supplying all the co-factors needed for bone synthesis, combined with a range of factors which are, broadly, anti-inflammatory/anti-erosion agents such as the flavonoids and isoflavones. And what are the key factors? There are many, but calcium and magnesium, although they are included, are relatively minor players.

Calcium and Magnesium

As osteoporosis develops, it is easy to detect that calcium and magnesium have been leached from the bones, and are being lost in the urine. From this humble finding, it was decided that the best way to remedy osteoporosis was to pump patients full of – yes – calcium and magnesium. The problem is that this approach is singularly ineffective. Even when vitamin D is added to the mix, the therapeutic effects are slight indeed. This is because calcium and magnesium are not the problem, but a symptom.

When you begin to lose minerals from your bones, it is as if the slates on your roof have started to fall off because the copper nails that hold them in place have rusted through. Taking huge doses of calcium and magnesium is like throwing pieces of slate up on to the roof, in the vain hope that they will stick there. That's patently stupid, when what is needed is a new set of nails. But what does this mean in terms of bone?

Vitamin K

When bone is re-modelled, pockets of old bone are eroded by cells called osteoclasts. These secrete one set of enzymes which dissolve the mineral salts, and another set which dissolve the microfibres; in other words, that specialized part of the extra-cellular matrix which acts as a template for the bone. Once the pocket of old bone has been dismantled, another set of cells arrives – the osteoblasts – whose function is to rebuild new bone where the old bone used to be. They start by secreting microfibres, forming a pre-mineralized form of bone called osteoid, and then they produce a protein called osteocalcin. This is activated by vitamin

K, and once activated it grabs calcium and magnesium from the extra-cellular fluids and plasma, locks them into place and the process of mineralization begins.[3] Gradually the soft osteoid becomes hard new bone, and the cycle is complete.

The bone has been renewed, and all is well, but as you can see, the calcium and magnesium are at the end of a long and complex assembly line. If the process that makes osteoid (the 'nails') is incomplete, and if there is insufficient vitamin K to activate the osteoid, all the calcium and the magnesium in the world will have little effect, as there is nothing to hold them in place.

Vitamin K – Best Sources

Traditional sources of Vitamin K include kale, Brussels sprouts and broccoli, although the fermented cheeses are better sources.

It's important to note that if you are taking an anti-K coagulant such as Warfarin for the prevention of blood clots you must not take extra vitamin K. Vitamin K reduces the effectiveness of the anti-coagulant which may lead to thrombus formation. Everyone else, however, can safely take vitamin K. In Japan osteoporosis patients routinely take up to 45 mg of vitamin K per day.

The problem, as ever, is Type B malnutrition – and most of you have this. In this situation the preliminary process of bone erosion proceeds too far and too fast, because the damping elements that should be present in the diet (flavonoids, isoflavones) are not there in anything like the correct amounts. Once the process of bone building begins, the osteoblasts cannot produce enough microfibres (because they are short of manganese, copper, zinc, vitamin C and the B vitamins, etc.), so inadequate amounts of osteoid are formed. When mineralization occurs, it too is hampered by lack of vitamin K, and so once the cycle of erosion and renewal has completed, there is a little less bone there than there was before. The cycling continues, and at every stage there is a little less bone made than there was eroded, until the bones are so thin that they fracture.

The Ideal Anti-Osteoporosis Supplement Programme

This should include 2 mg of manganese, 2 mg of boron, 2 mg of copper and 10 mg of zinc a day, together with vitamins K, D and B6. Include ipriflavone at 600–1,200 mg a day, glucosamine at 500–1,000 mg a day and calcium and magnesium at 600 and 300 mg respectively.

If you put a wide spectrum micronutrient support programme in place, you give your bones a better chance of cycling correctly, and maintaining their strength and integrity. And if you manage to do this, you will not need the absurdly high doses of calcium and magnesium currently in vogue. If the bone-building cells have all they need to make osteoid, and your diet contains enough vitamin K to allow the osteoid to mineralize, relatively little calcium and magnesium is needed. In fact, there is evidence emerging that the excessive doses of these two minerals currently recommended may increase the risk of certain cancers, due to their effects on vitamin D.

If you are female, you can always fall back on hormone replacement therapy (HRT). This may be a money-spinner for the drugs industry, but after a recent European review, the MHRA stopped recommending HRT as the first choice in protection against osteoporosis (MHRA Press Release, November 2003) due to growing safety concerns such as increased risks of stroke and breast cancer.[4]

Osteoporosis, just like osteoarthritis, vascular disease and most of the other chronic degenerative diseases, represents a system failure caused by multiple weak links, mostly caused by the lack of a range of key co-factors, vitamins, minerals or phytonutrients. As these system failures are due to the lack of many different micronutrients, attempting to rectify them with crudely fashioned pharmaceutical spanners is a strategy which cannot cure, and carries a high incidence of toxicity. For example, many osteoporosis drugs cause side-effects such as heartburn, abdominal pain, constipation, diarrhoea, irritation of the oesophagus and dysphagia (difficulty swallowing). This is exactly what modern medicine has given us. But by looking after your own health and by providing your body with what it needs to maintain itself, your risk of illness will be dramatically reduced, and your dependence on the current crisis-management model of medicine minimized.

If you don't care about your bones, maybe I should try to appeal to your vanity. How would you like to slow the ageing of your skin? The matrix comes in here too, because much of the appearance of skin is due to the integrity of the specialized extra-cellular matrix that underpins it, and provides it with strength, elasticity and moisture retention. Just as in cartilage and bone, the matrix here can be renewed. The next section shows you how.

Skin

When skin ages, there are really two quite different things going on. One is the loss of muscle mass and tone in the muscles underlying the skin, which leads to a general drooping of the skin and features, which is particularly apparent round the cheeks and jaw line. This can be largely rectified by the new muscle-stimulating systems such as Zenique (see page 161). The other is a series of changes to the texture of the skin itself, comprising a loss of plumpness and elasticity. And this can be stabilized using appropriate pharmaco-nutritional programming.

The plumpness and elasticity of the skin is largely determined by that part of the extra-cellular matrix that underlies the skin. The three-dimensional mesh of microfibres here includes the proteins collagen and elastin which provide tensile strength and elasticity respectively, and the glucosamine polymer hyaluronic acid, which determines the hydration capacity or plumpness of the skin.

The microfibres in the matrix in the skin turn over constantly, as they do in every other part of the body, but in the skin they are subject to an additional rate of attrition, due to exposure to ionizing radiation. Ultraviolet (UV) in sunlight penetrates the skin, and can kill cells outright (leading to peeling); cause cancer (in a small minority of cases) or simply damage the skin cells, leading to rupture of their cell membranes. When this happens the cells release a cloud of enzymes called matrix metallo-pro-teases, which break down all the fibres in the matrix under the skin. This causes inflammation (the reddening after excess sun exposure), and local breakdown of the matrix.

If you are well nourished, and the matrix is not under severe attack, skin only ages very slowly. Compare the skin of your under-arm, next to the arm pit – or indeed in any other area of your body where the sun don't shine – and you will see that it looks markedly younger than the skin on your face, neck and hands, which tend to be the most exposed areas. If you were to take small samples of the skin from the under-arm and the hand and put them under a microscope, they would show the same thing; even at the cellular level, ageing of the skin is very much slower in the sheltered areas, and dramatically accelerated in the exposed areas.

Of course, as you age you have to factor in the effects of Type B malnutrition. The body becomes progressively more depleted in protective factors such as the carotenoids, anti-inflammatory factors such as the flavonoids, and renewal and repair factors such as glucosamine, vitamin C, copper and zinc. Under these condi-tions the rate of damage to the matrix under the skin accelerates, and rates of repair and regeneration take a nose-dive. Not surpris-ingly, the matrix deteriorates. It becomes disorganized, less elastic, and physically thinner. As a result the skin cells become disorganized too, and the strength, elasticity, fineness and mois-ture-retaining ability of the skin all begin to fail.

Smoking, of course, accelerates skin ageing via a number of different mechanisms including excessive oxidation, 'curing' of the skin and deterioration of the capillary beds under the skin; three more reasons to get rid of that tobacco habit. And then there is glucose. A diet which contains excessive amounts of digestible carbohydrates pours too much glucose in the blood-stream and, as that kind of diet is usually low in the protective flavonoids, protein denaturation speeds up, not just in the kidneys and eyes, but in the skin also. This is a major component in the accelerated ageing of people with diabetes.

Skin ageing therefore mostly consists of excessive matrix breakdown. This in turn is largely caused by Type B malnutrition, which leads to excessive inflammation, excessive oxidative stress (smoking, excessive sun exposure) and excessive protein denaturation (diabetes). Once the complex process of skin ageing has been broken down into its constituent elements, however, it is relatively easy to stabilize the skin and reverse many aspects of the ageing process. Skin thickness and strength can be improved, wrinkles and fine lines reduced and eliminated. All these promises are already claimed by various cosmetic manufacturers, but a glance at the list of contents of their products tells you that they cannot achieve much. Stuck in the pharmaceutical mindset, most still cling to the idea that ageing is a linear process which can be alleviated with a single magic bullet. Neither of these ideas is accurate or true.

The Solution

Pharmaco-nutritional programmes designed to reverse skin ageing start from a different premise. Ageing is largely the result of a deterioration in the extra-cellular matrix, so the remedy must be to simultaneously slow the rate of any further matrix breakdown using micronutrients which absorb UV, mop up free radicals and block the tissue-damaging matrix metallo-protease enzymes; and speed the processes of repair, by supplying the body with all the myriad of co-factors it needs to regenerate the damaged matrix.

When such a programme is used on its own, it is reported to lead within two to three months to improvements in skin texture which many users describe as 'dewiness'. It has no effect on the underlying musculature, however, which limits its efficacy. On the other hand, electro-stimulation of the muscles (explained on page 161) improves facial muscle tone and the 'drape' of the face, but has little effect on skin texture. When the two approaches are combined, however, the effects are genuinely remarkable and, according to many of the subjects who volunteered for this somewhat experimental approach, habit-forming!

Skin Savers

Diet and exercise have a big impact on your skin. Here's your optimum programme for youthful skin.

- Ensure you are getting plenty of antioxidants, vitamins C and E, B vitamins, carotenoids, flavonoids and Q10 in your diet. A wide range of fruit and vegetables is an ideal place to start.
- Blackcurrants, blueberries and elderberries all contain matrix-stabilizing flavonoids, so make them a regular feature of your diet. Combine with glucosamine, manganese and betaine.

Cancer

Moving from vanity to fear, cancer and skin ageing turn out to have certain elements in common. In both cases, damage to the extra-cellular matrix is a key part of the process.

From the point of view of a cancer cell, life is hard. Cells in the body are becoming cancerous all the time, as a result of DNA mutations, but in the vast majority of cases, these cells either die spontaneously or are identified by the immune system and destroyed. A very small proportion of cancer cells manage to avoid these fates, and start to multiply, but are brought up short by the presence of other cells which have receptors on their surface that tell neighbouring cells with similar receptors to stop growing. The cancer cell stops, unless it finds a way to remove its inhibitor receptors.

A healthy diet contains a number of compounds which can force cancer cells to re-express their inhibitor receptors, and as soon as they do they must stop growing. Nevertheless, a small percentage of the cancer cells that have got this far manage to keep their inhibitor receptors under wraps, and continue to proliferate. Now, however, they run into a new set of restrictions; the extra-cellular matrix stands in their way, and holds them in place. The matrix also presents another problem because the cancer cells – now numbering several millions – need to find a blood supply or choke to death. They need to attract new blood vessels, but the omnipresent matrix presents a series of barriers to any capillary that would otherwise grow towards the developing tumour.

If the cancer is to progress, it must destroy the matrix so that a new blood supply can be achieved. The successful cancer cells now use another trick; they secrete the same group of matrix-destructive enzymes (the matrix metallo-proteases) as are involved in the ageing of skin, and which have the same result here. The matrix is punched full of holes, new blood vessels can grow in and the tumour really takes off. Even worse, the holes in the matrix allow metastasis, the process whereby cancer spreads from an original tumour via the lymphatic network and the bloodstream to other sites in the body.

Supplements to Provide an Anti-Cancer Shield

- a broad spectrum of vitamin/mineral antioxidants
- a flavonoid complex
- co-enzyme Q10
- betaine and occasionally echinacea
- a pre-biotic supplement
- mixed carotenoids for echinacea substitute yeast beta glucans

A healthy diet presents the cancer with many additional problems. Such a diet contains compounds which can kill many cancer cells, or force them to re-differentiate (revert to their former, non-cancerous forms). It will contain other compounds which block the matrix metallo-proteases, and stabilize the microfibres of the matrix, thereby blocking the ingrowth of blood vessels.

The healthy diet, according to the American National Cancer Institute, should contain at least nine portions of fruit and vegetables a day (women are let off with a slightly lower 'dose'). Very few people eat this amount of fruits and vegetables; in the UK, very few manage to meet even the UK government's less ambitious recommendations of five a day. And as we get older our intakes of fruits and vegetables, which are too low to start with, drop even further.

The increasing incidence and severity of Type B malnutrition in middle-aged and older people helps to explain why the incidence

Anti-Cancer Foods

The best foods to eat for a cancer-fighting profile are generally a wide range of fruit and vegetables. A number of culinary herbs also contain health-promoting nutrients.

- brassica vegetables such as kale, cabbage, Brussels sprouts and broccoli
- citrus fruits
- tomatoes
- green tea
- spinach
- rosemary, thyme, oregano and garlic
- onions
- soy products such as soy milk and soy beans
- wheat or rice bran
- walnuts
- raspberries, blueberries and blackberries
- turmeric
- pears
- shitake mushrooms.

The general principles of an anti-cancer diet are: more fruit and vegetables, more grains, pulses and legumes and fewer fats, sugars, salt and smoked or pickled foods.

of cancer increases as we get older. All the layered defences against the cancer cell are in a state of disrepair. The immune system, depleted in many of the micronutrients it needs in order to function properly, is faltering; the compounds that would normally keep cancer cells in check or kill them have gone; there is nothing to block the destruction of the extra-cellular matrix.

You can of course stay on your current bad diet, wait to develop cancer and then throw yourself on the tender mercies of the oncologist. I would rather eat a good diet, supplemented with the relevant micro- and phytonutrients, and stay healthier for longer.

CLAYTON PLAN TOP TIP 11

Baked Stuffed Mackerel (see Chapter 7) features many powerful antioxidants important for skin regeneration and fighting free radicals. Red wine is high in flavonoids, thyme and garlic are powerful antioxidants and leeks contain the flavonoid quercitin that neutralizes free radical action in the body.

NEW DIRECTIONS IN TOTAL HEALTH AND WELL-BEING

- New ways to quit smoking
- New ways to younger-looking skin
- Fat burning

11
New Ways to Stop Smoking

It's hard for smokers to give up their habit – and even harder if you are concerned, as many smokers are, that giving up leads to weight gain. So why do we smoke?

We smoke when we're bored, after a meal, when we're trying to concentrate, or relax, or perhaps because we have no other pleasure in life. But most smokers don't want to smoke. We're concerned about cancer, heart disease, the way the cigarette habit yellows our teeth and ages our faces. But we smoke because we're addicted to nicotine – and nicotine is a pervasive, persuasive drug. Many people who have been addicted to both heroin and tobacco have told me that of the two, tobacco is the harder to kick – because while you can leave heroin culture behind, tobacco is everywhere. And smoking, many people find, helps them to keep the weight off, so it's understandable that they worry about stopping if it means piling on the pounds.

The Effect of Nicotine

Nicotine acts in the brain by stimulating nerve receptors that are involved in transmitting certain types of information, and helping you to focus. Professor Keith Wesnes of Cognitive Drug Research, a world-leader in computer-based brain screening systems, has shown that very tiny doses of nicotine – which you can obtain by chewing the corner of a piece of nicotine gum – produce measurable improvements in mental tasking.

But the brain is very adaptive, and if you keep flooding the inside of your skull with nicotine these same receptors become less sensitive in order to compensate for all the drug-induced stimulation. Stop smoking, and the low-sensitivity receptors, no longer driven by nicotine, leave activity in this section of the brain slow and uncertain. This leaves you muzzy, unfocused, irritable and unable to concentrate.

This is exactly what scopolamine, the 'truth drug' does; it reduces the sensitivity of the same nerve impulses by blocking these same receptors. Professor Wesnes has shown that taking away a smoker's cigarettes leaves him or her in a state that exactly mirrors the effects of the 'truth drug'. It is no wonder that, once the last cigarette has been stubbed out and nicotine levels in the brain start to fall, the smoker soon starts to crave the next cigarette just to get his or her brain back up to speed.

Why Nicotine Patches Don't Work

Nicotine isn't exactly a health food, but it is the carbon monoxide, free radicals, tars and other combustion products in the smoke which do the damage that leads to the many diseases that smokers are so prone to. Hence the nicotine patch, which cleanly and safely dulls the craving for nicotine, and allows smokers to wean themselves painlessly off their habit. Except that patches don't work. The early trial results which seemed to show how very effective the patches were in helping smokers to give up were, it now appears, somewhat skewed, and presented in such a way as to promote the sales of these products. Initial enthusiasm was damped by subsequent less promotional trials. A well-designed English study in 2000, for example, revealed that after a year on patches only 10% of the original abstainers remain non-smokers – a rate hardly distinguishable from placebo.[1]

Patches don't work because they don't deliver the nicotine in a way that satisfies. The smoker gains a hit of nicotine with every drag, which produces a nicotine spike that enters the lungs, the bloodstream and finally the brain. The patch, on the other hand, delivers a slow, even trickle of the drug into the blood which, most smokers find, just doesn't hit the spot. Just as bad, patches gives no hand-to-mouth action, which is one reason why they are so poor at preventing weight gain in smokers trying to give up.

Nicotine Gum

Nicotine gum is an alternative way of taking the drug. Some prefer it to the patch because they can control their nicotine dosage rather more carefully, and find that chewing satisfies the oral urge. This makes the gum slightly more effective than patches, but not much. Long-term dependence can be a problem with this method, and a small minority of the ex-smokers who finally manage to kick the cigarette habit continue to chew the gum for years after they formally 'quit'.

In any case, the gum is not as easy to use as you might think. Patients starting to quit must chew one to two pieces each hour, but no more than twenty pieces a day. The gum must be chewed slowly until it develops a peppery taste. Then it must be stored between the gum and cheek so that the nicotine can be absorbed. Coffee, tea, soft drinks, and acidic beverages such as fruit juices can all interfere with nicotine absorption, so people have to wait at least 15 minutes after drinking before chewing a piece of gum.

Many people won't use the gum because it tastes frankly unpleasant, and can cause side-effects such as upset stomach, mouth ulcers and throat irritation. The latest generation of gums and films however, are much better in this respect, and are very helpful for smokers in situations where smoking is not allowed. Then there is the nicotine spray – helpful in dulling the immediate cravings but it can irritate the nose, eyes, and throat, and is not very effective except, possibly, among the nasally fixated – and the nicotine inhaler.

The Nicotine Inhaler

The inhaler looks pretty much like a plastic cigarette holder, but without the faded glamour. It comes with nicotine cartridges which must be inserted before the device can be used. The inhaler provides varying doses of nicotine on demand, as opposed to the patch or gum which supply nicotine in a drip-feed. What is more, the inhaler satisfies the oral (and hand-to-mouth) urges, which is probably why the success rates with this type of device are as high as 25%.[2]

The major problem with this system is that the particles delivered by the inhaler are so large that most of the inhaled nicotine is dumped into the mouth and not the airways. This is quite different from the cigarette, and can cause throat irritation in even hardened smokers.

Reduced-Smoke Cigarettes

A recent alternative is the R J Reynolds Eclipse, a so-called reduced-smoke cigarette. In this system the tobacco isn't actually burned at all. The smoker lights the tip of a carbon rod that runs down the middle of the cigarette, separated from the leaf by a glass-fibre sleeve, and effectively vaporizes the tobacco.

Eclipse cigarettes deliver nicotine in the same way that a normal cigarette does, which is why smokers like them; but, despite an intensive advertising campaign (in the US), health authorities remain very concerned.[3] Eclipse generates carbon monoxide, which is dangerous to the heart and, in one study,[4] levels of carcinogens such as the nitrosamines, acrolein and benzo(a)pyrene were often much higher than in low-tar cigarette brands. Another potential danger with Eclipse is that the glass insulating fibres could become dislodged and inhaled into the lungs. Their carcinogenic effects in the lungs may be similar to asbestos fibres, but this is as yet unknown.

The R J Reynolds company defended its product, saying that Eclipse has been extensively tested and the results independently reviewed; however other bodies such as the American Cancer Society have called for the removal of Eclipse from the market place.

The Smoke and Tobacco-Free Cigarette

There is, however, a new and highly sophisticated system that delivers nicotine directly into the lungs, without smoke – or, indeed, tobacco. This is the Aerocel, which uses controlled chaos and exquisite flow mechanics to produce a spray of nicotine particles that are uniformly between 0.5 and 2 microns (millionths of a metre) in diameter. Particle size is critically important. Smaller particles are breathed in, then out again, and are lost. Larger particles are deposited in the mouth and throat, leaving a bad taste and irritation, and never reach the lungs at all. But particles in the 0.5 to 2 micron range pass deep into the airways and down into the alveoli where they deliver nicotine directly and rapidly into the bloodstream – just as cigarette smoke does.

A single hand-held system, shaped like a cigarillo, contains enough nicotine to stand in for a packet of 20 and will retail in a broadly similar price band. It satisfies just as cigarettes do, and furnishes all the hand-to-mouth coordination that any smoker could wish for. There is no unpleasant taste or irritation of the throat – in fact, it is effectively a cigarette without the carbon monoxide, and without the carcinogens and free radicals. Another key advantage is that as there is no smoke, there are no passive smokers; clean nicotine can be used in company without offending bystanders, or putting them at risk. It can be used in no-smoking areas, and even on flights.

The Aerocel has not yet been tested in terms of its ability to help smokers give up, and it is, frankly, likely to be just as addictive as cigarettes. But if I was a smoker and could not give up the habit, I would switch to this system immediately to reduce my risk of smoking-related disease. And I would not be concerned about weight gain as there would be no nicotine withdrawal symptoms, and there would be no oral compensation needed.

The only problem will be if you live in the European Union. Although these Aerocels will be sold in the Americas and in the Middle and Far East by mid-to late 2006, Brussels will almost certainly deem them to be too radical for Europeans to use. This means that we will have to go on dying of tobacco-related diseases in large numbers, or buy them over the internet.

CLAYTON PLAN TOP TIP 12

Smokers need extra supplements of vitamins and minerals to repair the damage done by cigarettes. Ensure you're obtaining these either through your diet or, more reliably, via supplements. We know that life and dietary habits can reduce the risk of tobacco-induced illness. For example, the French smoke as much or more than the British or Americans, yet suffer less heart disease, due, it is thought, to a healthier diet and higher levels of physical activity.

12
The Knife-less Facelift

As the years pass, and even if we have virtuously maintained our body weight, our faces start to betray the passage of those years. This can be particularly evident in those who have lost substantial amounts of weight, and in smokers, sun-worshippers and the poorly nourished. In our vain and competitive times, the desire to turn the clock back has made aesthetic surgery one of the most lucrative medical specialities. Women and men now routinely buy new eyes, noses, jawlines and waistlines, thanks to the twin miracles of non-reactive implants and liposuction.

The writing, however, is on the wall. Antibiotic resistance is fast gaining ground in the hospitals and in the community, making even the most powerful antibiotics redundant. You could place some of the blame for this on doctors for over-prescribing; but don't forget the vast veterinarian grey market in antibiotics (where antibiotics are smuggled across borders); the indiscriminate use and over-the-counter sales of antibiotics in many less well-regulated countries; the failure of many patients to take their prescriptions properly and their demands for antibiotics even when they are not necessary.

The result may be that soon the antibiotics will not be effective when we really do need them. There was a time – in living memory, for anyone over the age of 80 or so – when any minor cut or scratch could be lethal if you were unlucky enough to develop septicaemia, or blood poisoning. There were no adequate treatments until 1935, when first the sulphonamides and then the penicillins brought the infectious diseases under control, and laid the foundations for the modern era of allopathic medicine.

Would we have developed vanity surgery if every procedure, from an eyelid lift to dermabrasion, carried a significant risk of infection and death? Is a better profile worth facing death for?

This is not just a theoretical question. For many clinicians and microbiologists the question is not whether the age of antibiotics is going to end, but when. Warning bells – such as recent reports of the dangerous antibiotic-resistant strains MRSA (methicillin-resistant *Staphylococcus aureus*) and VRSA (vancomycin-resistant *Staphylococcus aureus*), the so-called 'super-bugs' coinciding in the same London hospital – have still not been understood by the public, though they herald the beginning of the end.

There are already many problems associated with aesthetic surgery. The results can be unpredictable and, in the hands of the wrong surgeon, disfiguring. It is expensive, swelling and bruising round the operating site can take weeks or occasionally months to fully resolve, there may be excessive scarring. As we continue to run out of antibiotics the rising risk of infection will undoubtedly check the runaway development of this medical speciality, and will make lifesaving surgery very difficult too.

By great coincidence, we are now entering the era of knife-less cosmetic enhancement. There is a pioneering new British technology called Zenique which offers an alternative to cosmetic surgery, and it is based on a new understanding that facial ageing consists of two different processes, each one of which can be stabilized and at least partly reversed.

One of these is a deterioration of the extra-cellular matrix (described on page 134), a three-dimensional mesh of microfibres that gives the skin elasticity and strength and allows it to remain hydrated. This deterioration is a complex process that involves a balance between the rates of skin regeneration on the one hand, and the rates of breakdown on the other. The balance is tipped towards breakdown by Type B malnutrition, by exposure to excess sunlight, and by smoking. Both the regeneration and the breakdown side of the equation can be modified, using pharmaco-nutrition; the recipe for this approach to reversing skin ageing is given in Chapter 10.

The other major process that contributes to the ageing of the face is the gradual loss of tone and tension in the muscles and tendons that lie under the skin, and hold it in place. And this process is, it now turns out, surprisingly easy to modify and to reverse.

Facial Exercise

The idea of facial exercises as an anti-ageing strategy is as old as the hills, and works reasonably well for those dedicated enough to do the exercises on a daily basis. The regime is time-consuming, however, and makes you look frankly ridiculous – try doing the exercise routine in front of your partner! Various electronic devices are sold for home use which claim to stimulate the deep muscles, but these are ineffective because the voltage needed to access the deep muscles causes too much discomfort if surface (skin) electrodes are used. The standard stimulators routinely combine surface electrodes with a 9 volt battery, which tells you that they cannot do more than make the skin tingle. This may feel therapeutic, but achieves nothing. The only way these devices could work would be if the electrodes were driven through the skin and inserted directly into the muscles, a painful and invasive procedure which you should not try at home.

The goal – to achieve deep muscle stimulation with surface electrodes, but without the pins and needles – has until now proved impossible. The new Sigma Q technology from Zenique solves that old problem using an ingenious approach. It uses sophisticated electronic switching and gating systems to provide, instead of a single large charge (which stimulates the sensory nerves and causes the pins and needles), a series of micro-charges at rates of up to 20,000 per second which bypass the sensory nerves altogether. Once a series of micro-charges has been delivered, the switching system breaks the circuit, and as there is now no return path to the generator for the charge it has no alternative but to dissipate via the path of least resistance – which is muscle tissue. The result is a profound stimulation of the muscles via their motor nerves with little if any stimulation of the sensory nerves, and no pins and needles.

Medical versions of this equipment are already being used in hospital neurology departments and pain clinics in Britain and the US to treat neuropathies such as Guillain-Barré Syndrome. They are also being used by osteopaths, physiotherapists and sports rehabilitation specialists to treat tennis elbow, frozen shoulder and a variety of other difficult and painful conditions.

At the time of writing Zenique was due for release for cosmetic applications in the High Street hair and beauty salons in 2005, in Europe, the US and Japan, under the tag line 'Send your face to the gym'. Having tried one of these machines, I can vouch that the feeling after a session with this system is exactly that, the same muscle glow that you get after a workout at the gym, all over the face. It's an odd but pleasant feeling.

In the trials that I observed, I noted that after three or four thirty-minute sessions the face starts to change. The improving muscle tone lifts the features quite dramatically, filling out lines and removing, for example, the sag under chin and cheeks. Interestingly, there is some preliminary evidence that at specific stimulation frequencies, the fat cells that fill out the bags under middle-aged and elderly eyes begin to break down, a phenomenon called lipolysis, and are gradually resorbed. The combined effect on the eye of toning the orbital muscles and apparently removing the fat cells resembles, in several cases I have seen, the effects of an eye lift *and* eye bag removal, or an upper and lower blepharoplasty.

So now that you've dieted, exercise and toned, and look and feel 20 years younger, what are you going to do with it?

CLAYTON PLAN TOP TIP 13

To save your skin make the following foods a regular part of your diet: blackcurrants, bilberries, elderberries and green tea. They are rich in beneficial flavonoids, which block tissue-destructive enzymes. Drinking half a litre of soy milk has an additional protective effect.

13
Natural Viagra

Sexuality and health are connected in many different ways. Promiscuous and unprotected sex can, of course, be distinctly hazardous, but neuropsychologist Dr David Weeks, head of the Old Age Psychology Department at the Royal Edinburgh Hospital, and others have shown that in general, carnality and longevity go together.

There are several possible explanations for this. Dr Weeks suggests that it may be that sex promotes good health by, for example, stimulating the release of growth hormone. An alternative explanation is that as we get older, it is only the healthier elderly people who are still capable of having sex. In fact, both these explanations are probably partially true.

Undoubtedly, however, general health affects sexual appetite and performance. And undoubtedly, also, the incidence of erectile dysfunction – it affects 1 in 3 men at the age of 40, 2 in 3 men by the age of 70, and 3 million men in the UK in total – tells us that the majority of middle-aged and elderly men are not particularly healthy.

This is pretty much in line with American data that shows that by the time we enter our sixth decade, 5 out of 6 of us will have the symptoms of one or more of the chronic degenerative diseases.

Causes of Erectile Dysfunction

Erectile dysfunction is not always, however, a sign of an underlying disease. It can have many causes. It is often linked with anxiety arising from the misconception that sexual activity must lead to penetrative intercourse and ejaculation. When this expectation is unmet, many men consider the sexual act a failure – and men with this expectation are particularly vulnerable to anxieties and self-fulfilling prophesies of failure. Sexual counselling is the most appropriate form of treatment in these cases; and can often alleviate problems due to anxiety, stress and marital conflict.

Impotence is also a common side-effect of many drugs, including medicines such as anti-hypertensives, hormones, anti-depressants, tranquillisers, and some cold and flu remedies, and recreational drugs such as alcohol, tobacco, heroin and cocaine. In medical cases a change of prescription may sometimes be sufficient to cure the problem. Where recreational drug use is involved, rehabilitation or other support is indicated.

In middle-aged and elderly men, however, most cases of erectile dysfunction have an organic cause, specifically vascular disease and neurological disease. If either the blood vessels that supply the penis or the nerves that connect to it are below par, an erection is difficult or impossible to achieve and maintain. As diabetes damages both blood vessels and nerves, and the condition is increasing at an alarming rate, it is hardly surprising that impotence in ageing men is an increasingly common problem – and that prescription and 'grey' sales of Viagra and its competitors, Cialis and Levitra, are doing well.

Viagra and Similar Drugs

All these drugs act by blocking the enzyme PDE-5, which relaxes the blood vessels that supply the penis and increases blood flow and engorgement during sexual stimulation. They are helpful for many men, although the reported side-effects, including headache and indigestion, are a problem for some, and deaths have been reported, especially when Viagra is combined with nitrates.[1]

The success of these drugs, paradoxically, has given the old folk remedies a new lease of life. Once dismissed as fantasy, the science behind Viagra has shown us that there are indeed switches in the male metabolism which can be activated biochemically to improve erection quality. This leads to a very obvious question: do any of the traditional herbal remedies actually work?

Chinese Herbal Remedies

One remedy called Libidfit or Libex certainly does. The first product of its kind to be vetted by the SATCM (the Chinese state agency set up in 1987 to oversee traditional Chinese medicines), this contains standardized extracts of a number of herbs that have been used in China to improve male sexual performance since the seventeenth century. In 1998, the formula was shown in a Beijing University study to improve sexual function in over 90% of men with erectile problems.[2]

This is a spectacularly high figure, especially when you compare it with the 60% success rates claimed for the pharmaceutical products on sale in the West. One reason for this is that the drug companies think of the erection as a purely hydraulic problem, and that using a simple and specific drug that opens the lock-gates is an appropriate strategy. The Chinese, on the other hand, have long known that sex is a complex process, and it starts in the head. For this reason they have included in their formulation herbs that, like Viagra, contain compounds that block PDE-5 and relax the blood vessels that supply the penis. But they have combined these with other herbs that appear to act on dopaminergic nerves in the brain; nerves that are involved in the mysteries of excitement and desire.

It is this intoxicating combination of increased arousal and performance that has been reported to make Libidfit the world's first apparently genuine aphrodisiac. The 90% plus figure recorded in Beijing agrees pretty much with a recent Belgian trial, and the informal findings of andrologist Dr Ken Purvis, whose Oslo clinic is specially set up to measure and treat erectile dysfunction.[3]

Libidfit's duration of action is up to 18 hours, and as it does not rely on PDE-5 inhibition, and indeed does not block the enzyme completely, it has a relatively low incidence of the side-effects typical of this group of drugs. Changes in blood pressure, for example, have not been reported, although we must wait for large-scale clinical trials for a definitive picture.

This herbal product is already in wide use as a sexual enhancer, but has a genuinely therapeutic role in middle-aged and elderly men with erectile dysfunction. Having said all this, it is also the case that if men looked after themselves more effectively, maintained a healthy body weight, ate a better diet, smoked less or not at all, and took a reasonable amount of regular physical activity, most of them would have little or no need of it.

It is also true that over-the-counter products like Libidfit are not entirely free of problems. Erectile dysfunction can be a symptom of diabetes and coronary artery disease, conditions which are often not diagnosed until very late in the day. It has been suggested that if men went to their GPs complaining of erectile difficulties, this might alert the doctor to diagnose the underlying condition, in the same way that opticians often diagnose diabetes or hypertension during occular examinations. Men who self-medicate for their erectile problems, therefore, would be missed.

In the real world, unfortunately, many – perhaps most – men do not talk to their GPs about impotence; and many GPs are not yet as familiar with the idea of erectile dysfunction as a diagnostic as they should be. Basic screening involving taking a proper case history, and testing blood pressure and urinary glucose, would be more effective in picking up early cases of diabetes and vascular disease.

In any case treatments for erectile dysfunction are available to all via the web, and so the stable door – if not the bedroom door – is more or less wide open.

Although Libidfit is a natural and traditional remedy, and its active ingredient is quite distinct to Viagra, the Viagra patent is so all-encompassing that some patent lawyers are arguing that this 400-year old remedy belongs to Pfizer! The debate continues . . .

The Female Perspective

There is no exact equivalent to erectile dysfunction in women but impaired sexuality is often reported by women as well as by men. Local vascular engorgement is a part of the female sexual response, which led Pfizer to test Viagra in women, but the only effect was an increased number of headaches. This was fairly predictable – there is obviously a lot more to female sexuality than changes in local blood flow – and in any case the problem (from the woman's point of view) is generally not vascular at all, but a lack of sexual desire.

Sexuality is a complex and sensitive thing, and the lack of desire may have a number of different causes. Partnership difficulties often manifest themselves in bed. There could be psychosexual problems, but where a relationship is otherwise working well, the problem may be rooted in the body rather than the mind.

Some cases of reduced libido have medical causes. Thyroid insufficiency, for example, can reduce the libido to almost nothing. Treat the underlying medical malfunction and the symptoms, including the sexual ones, disappear.

Hormonal changes associated with the menopause are a more common cause of low libido, and are often reversed by HRT or, reportedly,[4] the isoflavones from plant sources such as soy. But it's not just oestrogen; other libido-determining hormones in women, as well as in men, include testosterone, noradrenalin and dopamine.

The Romans knew (empirically) about testosterone. It is said that they served meat dishes made of bulls' testicles at the start of their orgies, and today, both men and women with flagging libidos are sometimes treated with testosterone patches.

Various herbal equivalents are available on the net; it is unclear whether they are effective, as information about them is scarce or non-existent at the time of writing.

CLAYTON PLAN TOP TIP 14

Your sex drive is regulated by various hormones including oestrogen, progesterone and testosterone. To ensure these are properly balanced make sure you're getting adequate levels of vitamin B3 (niacin), vitamin B5, vitamin A, beta carotene, zinc and manganese or take a well-designed multiple micronutrient support programme.

14
New Ways to Burn Fat

As well as the well-worn duo of diet and exercise, there is a third way of losing weight; by increasing the rate at which the body 'burns' calories. Every body has an idling speed, as measured by the numbers of calories per hour it burns just to maintain life, and this is termed the basal metabolic rate or BMR. This is the rate at which you burn calories when watching TV, remote control in hand to prevent the over-exertion of having to walk over to the set to change channels. These calories are needed to keep all your cells and systems ticking over, and of course to keep you warm, at around 98.6 °F or 37 °C.

BMR can be roughly calculated by multiplying your weight in pounds by 10 (or your weight in kilograms by 4.5). If you weigh 140 lb your BMR will be close to 1,400 calories per day. To this you need to add enough calories to fuel any and all physical exertion. In a physically active culture this can be anything between an additional 1,500 and 2,500 calories per day. In our mechanized society, however, physical activities require on average a mere 600 calories per day. This takes us up to the average total calorific requirement of around 2,000 calories per day.

If you are a very sedentary person, two hours a day of physical activity could increase the numbers of calories you burn by up to 30%; for an average person, the increase would be smaller, at around 12–15%. But for the terminally lazy, there is another way of losing weight, namely by persuading the body to increase its BMR. In theory, at least, this could be done by turning up the thermostat, increasing your core body temperature, losing more heat, and thereby increasing the rate at which stored energy (fat) is burned to generate that heat. This approach is known as thermogenesis.

Thermogenesis has been rather discredited by supplement manufacturers who sell a variety of compounds claiming to be 'thermogenic'. Green tea, chilli peppers and many other compounds, which produce a slight increase in body temperature when force fed in massive doses to mice, have no effect when given in trace amounts to humans. Theophylline, ephedrine, caffeine and guarana are ineffective too, unless taken in near-toxic doses.

There is, however, a novel way of increasing your basal metabolic rate that is nothing to with what you put in your mouth – and everything to do with what you put on your back. It operates by activating a tissue or organ you probably didn't even know you possessed, called brown adipose tissue (BAT) or just plain brown fat.

Brown Fat

In the December 1993 issue of the science journal *Nature*, Dr Bradford Lowell, Professor Jean Himms-Hagen and colleagues reported a series of experimental findings that really started a new chapter in the science of weight control. They were studying the role of BAT in mice.

Mice have a patch of brown fat just between their shoulder blades. The Himms-Hagen team found that when BAT in mice is switched off (see page 174), the animals become more sensitive to the cold, their appetite increases and they get very fat. When the BAT is switched back on, all these changes go into reverse; the mice become better able to survive in the cold, their appetites decrease and their normal body weight is restored.

At this point a number of earlier scientific papers from many authors and many labs, which had presented all sorts of seemingly unrelated data, began to make sense. According to the textbooks, BAT occurs in small mammals and in human babies – but not in adults. But back in 1979, pioneering British researchers Dr Nancy Rothwell and Professor Michael Stock published a report in *Nature*, suggesting that men and women probably possess brown fat in areas such as the back, breastbone and neck that can be switched on when they eat excess calories.

One of the first to see the potential importance of BAT to weight loss was the independent scientist Nicholas Dynes Gracey, who first patented BAT-enhancing clothing as far back as 1986, and who now regards BAT as not merely a thermogenic organ, but a stress-adaptive tissue. But I digress. . .

Our bodies contain many different kinds of fat. A proportion of this consists of specialized phospholipids, which make up cell membranes and the insulating sheaths which lie around the nerves, essential for their normal function.

Most body fat is white fat, a sluggish and bulky tissue which stores excess calories, and increases our waist size. But we also have small amounts of brown 'stress-adaptive' fat which can be very metabolically active indeed; under certain conditions it starts soaking up lipids and glucose from the bloodstream, and oxidizing them to generate large amounts of heat. To put it crudely, white fat is the insulation, and brown fat is the boiler in which it can be burned. Babies have brown fat, but until recently most doctors thought it disappeared as we grow older.

Finnish Discoveries

That idea, however, is changing. Dr Pirkko Huttunen, Vice-President of the International Society for Adaptive Medicine, studied indoor and outdoor workers in northern Finland where, apart from a brief summer, the climate is usually cool or cold. To be more accurate she studied dead workers as at that time, in 1980, the only way of locating brown fat in the body was by dissection.[1]

Indoor workers had no discernible brown fat, and neither did outdoor workers who had died during the summer months. Those who died during the autumn and winter, however, had pockets of brown fat in the neck, around the base of the great vessels that supply the head and brain.

The most logical explanation is that the body adapts to cold by growing islands of brown fat in areas of exposed skin which allow the body to rev up its 'central heating', burning blood fats and sugars at increased rates to maintain body temperature.

Back in the Ice Age, brown fat must have been essential. How else could we have kept warm enough to live through the long glacial winters? But nowadays office jobs, central heating and warm clothing ensure that our bodies are seldom exposed or cold enough to stimulate the growth of brown fat, so the brown fat we have as babies usually fades away. This explains why so few other scientists have found brown fat in adults. Basically, we need to exercise to train our brown fat.

In the cold climate of the Ice Age we would have done that naturally; as autumn turned to winter and the temperature started to fall, the cooling would have switched on our brown fat automatically, preparing us for the cold winter months. This is exactly what we still see in animals. Healthy rats, for example, kept at a cool 4 °C (39 °F) increase the amount of brown fat between their shoulders after only a few days of chill, to increase their ability to generate heat and stay warm.

The Brown Fat Advantage

Brown fat is different from white fat in several ways. It has a much richer blood supply, and the fat cells are packed with dark mitochondria which give the brown fat its distinctive colour. Mitochondria are the small, bean-shaped structures inside cells where energy from the food we eat is 'burned' or oxidized to produce ATP, the energy molecule we use inside our cells, and heat. Every cell in our bodies contains mitochondria, but the mitochondria in brown fat are unique. Whereas mitochondria in other tissues are very efficient in producing ATP and generate heat almost as a by-product, the mitochondria in brown fat are set up to burn calories, and produce heat instead of producing ATP.

And they do so very effectively. Professor George Bray of the Pennington Biomedical Research Center in Louisiana found that certain stimuli cause the body to start heating up, and he and his team are convinced that brown fat is involved. Professor Bray stated: 'We are becoming aware that brown fat has a very specialized function. Even though there's not much brown fat in a typical adult, probably less than 1% of the body by weight, when it gets revved up it produces as much heat as the rest of the body combined.'[2]

Revving Up Brown Fat

So how do we get our brown fat 'revved up'? Do we have any of this highly metabolically active tissue? And where in our bodies is it lurking? Answers to these questions were provided by Stéphane Krief, Daniel Ricquier and their colleagues at the University of Paris.[3] Their team showed that in adults and children, small numbers of brown fat cells can be identified nestling deep inside deposits of white fat. In other words we all have a few, but they are in the main quiescent. Even more interestingly, the scientists found that when white fat cells are stimulated in certain ways they transform into brown fat cells, becoming more vascular and increasing their numbers of mitochondria.

Krief and Ricquier likened this to the changes that occur in muscle during training; it too becomes more vascular, and grows more mitochondria, so that it can work harder. But instead of physical exercise, they used caffeine or nicotine to trigger the shift from white to brown fat. This gives a new insight into the tense, chain-smoking and coffee-drinking types who stay skinny, but this is not a reason to get out the cigarettes or even, unless you like very strong coffee, the coffee grinder. There are other ways. . .

Quite early on it became apparent that brown fat was innervated; that is, there is a special group of nerves that supplies the brown fat cells, and has the ability to switch them on. These are sympathetic nerves, and are part of the sympathetic nervous network whose main role is as a sort of emergency system.

Whenever we are threatened or stressed, the sympathetic nervous system plays a crucial role. It is an essential part of the fight or flight response. When confronted with a dangerous or stressful situation the brain, albeit indirectly, fires up the sympathetic nerves. They speed up the heartbeat and increase the amount of blood it pumps; they close the arteries leading to the gut and open those feeding the muscles, so that they will be given more oxygen and be able to work more effectively; they stimulate the liver to produce glucose, so that the muscles will have the fuel they need. The platelets in the blood become more sticky, so that if you happen to be wounded in the ensuing conflict your on-board puncture repair kit will be in top form. And your sense of pain diminishes, so that in the heat of battle you will not be distracted by the discomfort of an ingrowing toenail or disabled by a non-fatal wound. (A variety of other interesting things happen besides, but this is not a physiology textbook so I will not go into them here.)

Now it seems that the sympathetic nervous system was also involved, back in the times when humans were evolving, in readying our bodies for winter. It reacted to the stress of cooling temperatures late in the year, and activated our brown fat so that when the cold came, we could still function. And this makes perfect evolutionary sense of Pirkko Huttunen's findings that we only grow significant amounts of brown fat in winter, and only when we are exposed to the cold.

Our Hunter-Gatherer Past

Brown fat is a very extravagant tissue, and would only be used when it was needed. Cast your mind back tens of thousands of years ago and imagine how life must have been when we were hunter-gatherers, living in caves. Food is not always available, calories have to be used efficiently. During the summer months when living is relatively easy, there is more food around so our ancestors eat what they can, putting on weight, storing energy for the lean times ahead both in their white fat, and as dried foods to be hidden away for later use. There is no need for brown fat now, the weather is warm enough and to burn calories for heat would be unhelpful and wasteful.

Autumn arrives, and while our ancestors can still find game and plant foods such as nuts and berries, the growing chill tells them that winter is coming. Food is getting scarcer, and they have to survive both scarcity and the gathering cold. Brown fat is slowly growing, and gradually becoming active. Now they can keep warm enough to survive the cold, and forage and scavenge for whatever food is still be found. Gradually they are burning off the calories stored in their white fat; if they had stored 15 kg (33 lb) of white fat during the summer and autumn, this would provide around 135,000 calories. Providing they have laid up enough food to last the winter, they are carrying inside their own bodies enough fuel to keep them warm until spring comes again. White fat is the fuel, and brown fat is the furnace they will burn it in.

Many thousands of years pass, and we return to the twenty-first century. Food is no longer scarce – in fact, agri-business has made food more available and cheaper than ever before. Designed as we are to survive the lean times, our psychology and physiology are overloaded by the contemporary culture of excess. Obesity and overweight are now so prevalent that they have become one of the most important causes of ill health and death. In this context, it is hardly surprising that the drug companies are trying to develop drugs which would achieve weight loss by persuading white fat cells to become brown fat, and to start burning calories. Such drugs are called thermogens, and they are probably not far off.

Thermogens

At the University of Ancona, Saverio Cinti and his colleagues have managed to transform white fat cells in rats into brown fat cells using a thermogenic drug with the catchy name of CL 316243.[4] CL 316423 acts by stimulating a receptor found in fat cells, called the beta-3 adrenoreceptor. When this is stimulated, it instructs the white fat cells to evolve into brown fat cells. As they do so they grow more mitochondria, and start to produce a protein called uncoupling protein 1, or UCP-1. UCP-1 has only one known function: it 'uncouples' the mitochondria in brown fat cells so that instead of making ATP, they make heat.

Other researchers had already shown that when CL 316243 is given to obese mice they lose weight and, as beta-3 adrenoreceptors also exist in humans, there is every reason to believe that drugs which work in this way would help us to lose weight too. Furthermore, their mode of action is ideal, as all the weight loss occurs from fat and not from muscle.

But there is a tiny problem. The beta-3 receptors of rodents have a different structure from those of humans, and while CL 316424 works in mice, it does not work in men. A pharmaceutical treatment for people is some way off, as no one has yet developed a safe drug. The drug companies are racing to develop the first drug that will activate human beta-3 receptors without undue toxicity, but this could still be years away.

Other Ways to Kick Start Brown Fat

In the meantime, here is an alternative which you can use to stimulate your own beta-3 receptors, up-regulate your own brown fat and start burning off the white fat. And it is, actually, quite simple. A little bit of cooling will do the trick. Not too much, but just enough to activate your sympathetic nervous system.

When CL 316243 is described as a beta-3 adrenoreceptor agonist, this means that it works by stimulating a type of receptor that the sympathetic nervous system would normally stimulate. In other words, it is mimicking one aspect of sympathetic nervous function; beta-1 and beta-2 receptors are also switched on by the sympathetic nervous system, elsewhere in the body, and drugs designed to stimulate beta-2 receptors are commonly used in the management of asthma. But how do we activate our sympathetic nervous systems to achieve the beta-3 response? How cool do we have to be, and for how long? And do we have to cool our whole bodies, or just certain parts?

Think of a modern central heating system. The location of the boiler is not that critical, but the position of the temperature sensor certainly is. You don't put it next to the boiler, or the system would be constantly switching itself off. And if you put the sensor in the cellar, the boiler would be on permanently. You put it, instead, in the most important place, which is the living area. The same principle holds in human heating.

Your Brain as Temperature Gauge

Of all the organs the brain is the most temperature-sensitive. If its temperature drops by even a degree, cognitive efficiency is impaired. As the temperature of the brain falls further our judgement fails, our thinking degenerates and we lose consciousness. From a design perspective, therefore, we would locate the temperature sensors next to the brain and the blood vessels that supply it, so that any drop in brain temperature would be enough to start the brown fat firing up.

This is more or less what the evidence suggests. There does indeed appear to be a population of nerves with specialized temperature-sensitive endings that lie below the skin around the base of the brain, down the back of the spine, and in the neck. Various studies indicate that when these nerve endings are cooled, the nerves send a message to the hypothalamus in the brain, instructing it to raise the thermostat. The brain then instructs the brown fat via the sympathetic nervous system to burn fuel, generate heat, and raise the brain and body temperature back up to normal.

Critically, using modern and highly sensitive techniques, scientists have recently found[5] significant amounts of brown fat in the necks of adults and children. This means that when brown fat becomes active, one of the first organs it warms is the brain, followed by the rest of the body.

This model explains why some people (typically nervous, stressful types) can overeat and remain slim; their brown fat enables them to shed excess calories rather than store them as adipose tissue. It also helps us to understand why others eat sparingly, yet still put on weight; it may be that they are simply not as good at burning off calories as heat because their brown fat is inactive, and must therefore store them as white fat. This could be why older people tend to put on weight, because with ageing brown fat becomes less efficient, and less able to burn unwanted calories.

It could also shed some light on why a tendency to overweight often runs in families. After height, BMI is the second most heritable body feature, and between 30% and 70% of body size and shape is genetically influenced. A number of genes have been identified which are involved in weight control, and in a few cases, mutations in these genes have been shown to lead to increased body weight. In some cases, such as the gene *MC4R*, this is mediated by excess appetite, as the individual is not as sensitive to satiety as he or she should be. And in other cases, it is mediated by a relative inability to burn excess calories, indicating that the brown fat system is not working properly.

Exercising in Cold Conditions

For most of us, however, the way to up-regulate brown fat is to exercise regularly in a cool environment. Swimming is probably the best way of doing this, and has been shown to increase brown fat in several animal models. The take-home message therefore is:

Exercise regularly in cool temperatures to train your aerobic ability to generate your own warmth by exercising, put the thermal underwear back in cold storage, and save on those fuel bills by turning down the central heating. . .

The idea that a chilly dip could be good for health was supported recently by Professor Vijay Vir Kakkar, head of the Thrombosis Institute in London. Professor Kakkar published a series of papers which showed that a daily cold bath regime, which he calls thermoregulatory hydrotherapy, stimulated brown fat, boosted the immune system and improved the circulation.[6]

Spending Time in the Cooler

Regular cold bathing is an acquired taste which, although it might suit certain ex-public-school boys, is probably off-putting for most. There are less Spartan alternatives. At the AFRC Babraham Research Institute in Cambridge, Dr Joy Dauncey has been studying the effects of warm and cool environments on the metabolic rate.[7] She found that at a temperature of 22 °C (72 °F) (which is cool, but warm enough to minimize shivering), her experimental women subjects boosted their metabolism by as much as 10%. This important research proved that a slight cooling of the body may trigger the brown fat, and start it burning calories to help maintain body temperature.

In a separate but complementary series of studies at the University of Ottawa, Jean Himms-Hagen has been studying the subtle effects of animal housing temperatures on brown fat.[8] Her work has hinted that brown fat thermogenesis is reduced in the overclothed and overweight, and increased in the underclothed and underweight.

Professor Himms-Hagen's findings are supported by studies on metabolic responses of young men and women to cold stress, by researchers Andrews and Jackson at Trinity College, Dublin. They discovered that the more obese we become (especially women), the more our nervous system reduces heat output in response to cold and other forms of stress. According to Dr Fred Andrews, this effect could compound the problem of weight loss in obesity. So is there a comfortable way of increasing your metabolic response to stress if you happen to be overweight?

Different Kinds of Brown Fat

There is one more piece of the puzzle before we can arrive at the solution. That was provided by Dr Juliet Heaton at Trinity College in Dublin, who discovered that not all brown fat deposits act in quite the same way. Like Doctors Huttenen and Riquier, she found brown fat in all age groups from babies to adults aged 80 but, most importantly, her work suggests that the type of brown fat found at the skin's surface, for example between the shoulder blades, is the most sensitive to the activating effects of cool temperatures.

The pattern is complete. This suggests that if we stimulate the cold receptors which lie down the length of the spine, and allow the area between the shoulder blades to vent heat, this should activate brown fat in the area and start it turning calories into heat. The receptors can be challenged, and the heat allowed to leave, by not cladding the area in layers of clothing. The rest of the body, however, can be kept at a comfortable temperature, and all this can be achieved by wearing clothes that provide comfortable warmth but have a heat-transferring section or strip that runs down the backbone.

Cool Zone Clothing

This is the concept pioneered by Adrenalin Research, run by Nick Gracey and medical biochemist Trevor Gunn, who has been testing a range of CLOtherapy sportswear at the Hove Clinic in Sussex. The clothing has 'coolzones' sited over the armpits, backbone, breastbone, groin and neck. During exercise, these coolzones give the underlying cold-sensitive nerve endings an invigorating cool air massage, and provide for heat release by allowing any sweat to rapidly evaporate, providing more strategic cooling.

Adrenalin Research are also marketing CLOtherapy to assist weight control. For the overweight, exercising with local cooling is employed to encourage the growth of brown fat, speed the rate at which excess food is converted into heat and gently shed surplus white fat.

There are additional benefits which relate to brown fat's other function in the body, which is to help regulate blood chemistry. As brown fat becomes more metabolically active it drains fats and glucose out of the bloodstream, resulting in a significant lowering of plasma lipids and improved blood glucose control. This shift in blood chemistry is highly desirable, as it reduces the risk of Type 2 diabetes and vascular disease, including coronary artery disease and stroke. It might sound novel, but there is a historical precedent.

Before Banting and Best discovered insulin in 1921, there were two treatments for diabetes. One of these, the no-carb diet, was pioneered in the 1870s by the French physician Dr Bouchardat. He had noticed the disappearance of glycosuria in his diabetic patients due to the rationing of food in Paris when it was under siege during the Franco-Prussian War. It was hard to get patients to adhere to this sort of semi-starvation regime: in the 1880s and 90s, the Italian diabetes specialist Professor Catoni kept his patients under lock and key in order to get them to follow their diets.

The other method was combined exercise and cold exposure, a kill-or-cure approach that was practised in puritanical communities in the north of Scotland and Canada. Exercise increases the rate at which skeletal muscle soaks up glucose, thereby removing glucose from the bloodstream. Cold exposure, by activating brown fat, has the additional effect of lowering blood glucose – so this strenuous approach would undoubtedly have had an impact on those poor patients who survived such heroic treatment.

There is much more that can be done today to counter the adverse effects of diabetes, and the pharmaco-nutritional approach is described in Chapter 9.

But what about weight control through clothing? Does it work?

Does it Work?

I was initially sceptical, but agreed to try CLOtherapy training for a few months over the winter of 1994. I'm lean, and I didn't lose weight – but then again, I didn't want to. What did happen was that I started eating five or six square meals a day. I was ravenous, constantly eating, but my weight stayed exactly where it was. All the calories in the food I was eating were being burned up and converted to heat. My basal metabolic rate (see page 4) and body temperature increased to such an extent that I could no longer bear to sleep under a duvet, even on the coldest nights, and slept instead under a single sheet. Colleagues and friends remarked that I was hot to the touch, and asked if I had a fever – but I remained free of colds and flu throughout the winter.

At the end of this trial period I was photographed down at

the docks in Stockholm, in January, when the temperature was 11 °C below freezing with an additional wind chill factor of −3 °C. Asa Moberg from the Karolinska Institute who took the photos wore an eiderdown jacket and full cold weather clothing. I wore a fashionable outfit consisting of boxer shorts, boots, gloves and a hat. She started to complain of the cold before I did – and I'm no stoic. Remarkable? Ask the inhabitants of Stockholm. For many years before my experiment, and during my stay there, a well-known eccentric used to walk into the city centre everyday of the year, wearing only underpants. The moral is that you don't have to be mad to do this sort of thing.

There is as yet no trial evidence to support the use of CLOtherapy. However, on the basis of my experience with wearing an Adrenalin shirt over a period of five months, CLOtherapy training does make a difference. If you can control your appetite as you train your brown fat to go into action your excess white fat should gradually melt away, like the memory of an unpleasant dream. And if you can manage to down 225 g (8 oz) of red peppers every day, the effects may be greater still.

For a free newsletter about CLOtherapy visit the ADRENALIN.org website.

CLAYTON PLAN TOP TIP 15

> **Remember that exercise remains the best way to both lose weight and improve your health. Inactivity is more dangerous than just being overweight. It's as unhealthy as smoking 20 cigarettes a day, high blood pressure or high cholesterol.**

Conclusion

The Problem

The global problems of overweight and obesity are due to the fact that most of us take in more calories than we use, and this is caused by two factors. We live insufficiently physical lives, with energy requirements so low that our appetites cannot adapt properly, and living in today's cafeteria culture, we eat too many foods with an excessive calorie to micronutrient ratio.

The Remedies

We need to find ways of integrating more physical activity into our lives – whether this means walking part way to work, eschewing lifts and elevators, gardening or taking dance classes. And we need to change our eating habits, switching to foods with a reduced calorific density and a high micronutrient content.

In the near future the food industry will be doing more in this respect, producing ranges of familiar foods with enhanced micronutrient/calorie ratios. Look out for ingredients such as Litesse, HiMaize and Splenda (sucralose). Many food companies with an interest in quality foods are already looking at these and other functional ingredients.

In the meantime, and for those who prefer to prepare their own meals, there are a number of simple food choices which automatically create dishes with high micronutrient/calorie ratios, fermentable carbohydrates and a low glycaemic load. For those who want to take their nutrition and likely health prospects to the next level, a broad spectrum micro- and phyto-nutrient support programme would be a logical addition. Such programmes should include not only the currently defined vitamins and minerals but also appropriate levels of flavonoids, isoflavones, lycopene, lutein and glucosamine, at the very least. Other nutrients such as astaxanthin, betaine, Q10, acetylcarnitine, the galactolipids and the conditionally essential sugars and amino sugars are under review, and may well join the 'must-have' list as more data accumulates to support their inclusion.

The Prospects

If we can achieve real improvements in the lamentable state of the western world's nutritional status, significant improvements in public and personal health will inevitably follow. The widespread incidence of Type B malnutrition makes a major contribution to accelerated ageing and disease; rectifying Type B with better food choices and properly designed supplements will delay the onset of disease, and lead to improved life expectancy – as any vet could tell you.

Life extension will bring massive social and personal changes in its wake. If you know, for example, that you have an excellent chance of extending your healthy and functional middle years into the nineties or beyond, the impact of this knowledge on decisions about career structure, family planning, politics and pension plans will be profound.

Hospital wards and indeed whole hospitals will close – for the right reasons. The delivery point of most healthcare will shift from the surgery and pharmacy to the supermarket checkout.

Tomorrow's functional foods will have basic nutrition and health information on the label and more detailed information concealed in bar codes which you will access using hand-held bar-decoders, already in use in many supermarkets. For those with an unhealthy interest in nutrition, yet more information – clinical trials and such-like – will be available on websites that can be perused on the decoders, or on the computer at home.

In the next phase, information about the foods you purchase will be integrated with home-use diagnostic programmes, already widely available, and home-use diagnostic kits that measure levels of biomarkers in your blood, sweat, urine and breath. (A biomarker is a measurable characteristic of a biological system that changes in illness or in the run-up to illness, or upon exposure to physical or chemical damage.) And this in turn will be integrated into your online shopping programme, guiding your food choices so that the next time the supermarket delivers, it will be a range of products designed to satisfy your taste-buds *and* keep you healthy.

This will of course be optional, but as preventive health is so much cheaper than the current model of crisis-management medicine, the government will doubtless provide cash incentives to those who consistently make healthy choices, and keep their biomarkers in the green zone.

Another option will be to make your food/health profile available online to your GP, so that when – if – something starts to go subliminally wrong, the doctor will know about it at an incredibly early stage; early enough to vastly improve the effectiveness of treatment, and the quality of your life.

Hard to believe we could generate such substantial health gains in this way? Look no further than Finland, where dietary shifts over the last two decades have reduced the national blood pressure enough to cut the incidence of heart attacks and strokes in half. And that's just the beginning. . .

Appendix 1
A Broad-based Micronutrient Programme for Optimum Health

Supplement	Paul Clayton Recommended Supplement Level
Vitamin A	800 mcg
Vitamin C	500 mg
Vitamin D	10 mcg
Vitamin E	100 mg
Vitamin K	50 mcg
Vitamin B1	7.5 mg
Vitamin B2	7.5 mg
Niacin	15 mg
Pantothenic acid	15 mg
Vitamin B6	7.5 mg
Folic acid	200 mcg
Vitamin B12	6.75 mcg
Biotin	150 mcg
Selenium	150 mcg
Zinc	10 mg
Calcium	100–150 mg

Supplement	Paul Clayton Recommended Supplement Level
Magnesium	100–120 mg
Chromium	120 mcg
Copper	1 mg
Manganese	2 mg
Iodine	100 mcg
Molybdenum	100 mcg
Carotenoids	
Beta carotene	7 mg
Lutein	6 mg
Lycopene	5 mg
Zeaxanthin	100 mcg
Flavonoids	
Oligoproanthocyanidins	200 mg
Polyphenol complex	300 mg
Other	
Betaine	450 mg
Isoflavones	40 mg
Omega 3 (EPA/DHA)	600 mg
Resistant starches	8–10 g
Co-Q10	30–60 mg
Glucosamine	500 mg

Appendix 2
Glycaemic Load of Foods

The table below provides a list of common foods with their Glycaemic Load (GL) rating beside them. It has been drawn up by Professor Janette Brand-Miller at the University of Sydney. The GL rating is much more useful to you than the Glycaemic Index (GI) rating. The GI rating only tells you how quickly a particular carbohydrate raises blood sugar levels, not how much of that carbohydrate is in the food. For example, watermelon has a high GI value, but there is in fact not very much carbohydrate in the fruit, so the GL rating is relatively low.

A GL of 20 or more is high, 11–19 is medium and a GL of 10 or less is low. For optimum health and weight control you should choose foods with a lower GL rating. A quick glance at the table shows you that most fruit, vegetables and legumes have GL ratings on the lower end of the scale – combine this with their health benefits and it's easy to see why these foods should form the basis of our diet.

Food	Serving size in grams	Glycaemic Load Rating
Cakes, sweets		
Croissant	57	17
Sponge cake	63	17
Pancakes (buckwheat)	77	22

Food	Serving size in grams	Glycaemic Load Rating
Apple muffin (made with sugar)	60	13
Milk chocolate	50	14
Drinks		
Apple juice, unsweetened, cloudy	250	10
Carrot juice	250	10
Orange juice, unsweetened	250	13
Tomato juice, canned, no added sugar	250	4
Cola fizzy soft drink	250	16
Orange flavoured fizzy soft drink	250	23
Sports drinks	250	40
Breads		
Bagel	70	25
Baguette, white	30	15
Sunflower and barley bread	30	6
Wholemeal rye bread	30	8
White wheat flour bread	30	11
Rye kernel bread	30	5
Cereals		
Porridge made from rolled oats	250	13
Muesli, natural	30	10
Cornflakes	30	21
Wheat biscuits	30	13
Puffed rice cereals, crispies etc	30	22
Cereal grains		
Cous cous	150	23
Risotto (Arborio) rice	150	36
Long grain boiled rice	150	23

Food	Serving size in grams	Glycaemic Load Rating
Basmati rice	150	22
Brown boiled rice	150	18
Semolina, steamed	150	6
Bulgur wheat, boiled	150	12
Pasta and noodles		
Fettucine (egg)	180	18
Instant noodles	180	19
Rice vermicelli	180	22
Spaghetti, white, boiled 10 mins	180	21
Spaghetti, wholemeal, boiled	180	16
Vegetables		
Peas	80	3
Pumpkin	80	3
Beetroot	80	5
Carrots (raw)	80	1
Potato, boiled	150	14
Potato, mashed	150	18
French fries, frozen, heated in microwave	150	22
Fruit, uncooked		
Apple	120	6
Apricot	120	5
Banana	120	12
Cherries	120	3
Grapes	120	8
Orange	120	5
Peach	120	5
Pear	120	4

Food	Serving size in grams	Glycaemic Load Rating
Plum	120	5
Legumes		
Baked beans, canned	150	7
Black-eyed beans	150	13
Butter beans	150	6
Chick peas, dried and boiled	150	8
Haricot/Navy beans	150	12
Kidney beans, canned	150	9
Lentils, red, dried, boiled	150	5
Soya beans, dried, boiled	150	1
Dairy		
Milk, cow's, full fat	250	3
Yoghurt, reduced fat	200	7
Soy milk, reduced fat	250	8

Glossary

acetylcarnitine: a nutrient which helps to generate energy. It is available as a supplement and can be ordered over the internet.

adipose tissue: white fat that stores excess calories and is responsible for expanding waists and hips.

amino acids: the basic building block from which proteins are assembled.

amino sugars: a molecule which combines a sugar with an amino acid, e.g. glucosamine. These form the basic building blocks from which hyaluronic acid and many other micro-fibres in the extra-cellular matrix are assembled.

anti-glycosylants: substances that help impede the process of glycosylation.

antioxidant: an enzyme or substance capable of neutralising free radicals, which in excess, could otherwise cause damage to tissue.

astaxanthin: a carotenoid, like lycopene and lutein, derived from a red marine alga called *Haematococcus pluvialis*. This compound is linked to various health benefits, including improved fertility, and probably possesses some anti-cancer benefits.

atheroma: a fatty substance that can collect inside the lining of the arteries if a person has the wrong diet and/or smokes. This can lead to angina or a heart attack.

B-cell: immune cell involved in inflammatory conditions such as asthma and rheumatoid arthritis. 'Damping the B-cells down' is an anti-inflammatory activity.

betaine: otherwise known as trimethyl glycine. Betaine is an effective source of vital methyl groups, which are needed for many processes inside the body, such as the synthesis of RNA, DNA and phospholipids.

biomarker: a measurable characteristic of a biological system that changes in illness or in the run-up to illness. It may also change upon exposure to physical or chemical stresses.

blepharoplasty: a procedure to remove fat, along with excess skin and muscle, from the upper and lower eyelids.

blood sugar levels: levels of glucose in the blood.

brown adipose tissue: otherwise known as brown fat, so-called because of the high numbers of mitochondria it contains. Unlike white fat, this tissue is highly metabolically active, and converts excess calories into heat. Brown fat, however, is only present in small amounts in the body.

carcinogen: a substance that can cause cancer.

caries: dental decay.

cell membrane precursors: compounds which are built into the membranes of cells in our bodies.

cholesterol: a waxy fat which is an essential component of cell membranes. It can also be found in the blood, and is a precursor for steroid hormones and bile acids.

chondroblasts: cells that form cartilage.

complex carbs: sugar polymers including starches, which are large numbers of sugar molecules linked together.

conditionally essential sugars: sugars which are needed in the body and which we can normally produce enough of. In certain conditions, we may not be able to make enough of them in the body and thus it becomes essential to obtain them from our diet in order to safeguard or improve our health. These sugars include mannose, lyxose and other rare and special molecules.

diastolic blood pressure: when blood pressure is measured, two readings are produced – systolic and diastolic. They represent the highest and lowest pressure readings. The lower of the two tells us something about the state of the arterioles (or resistance vessels); an elevated diastolic reading generally reflects endothelial dysfunction.

DNA mutation: changes in the DNA of a cell which can, in certain cases, lead to a cancer.

dysphasia: a complete or partial loss of ability to speak, read, write and comprehend others.

dyspraxia: difficulty in planning and completing intended fine motor tasks.

EFA: essential fatty acids. These include omega 3 (as in fish oil) and omega 6 (as in many vegetable oils).

elastin: a protein micro-fibre that provides elasticity and is an essential part of the extra-cellular matrix.

endothelial dysfunction: chronic, sub-clinical inflammation of the blood vessels. In the small arteries, this causes constriction and an increase in blood pressure.

enzyme: a protein molecule made in the body, which acts as a catalyst for certain chemical reactions.

epidemiological: related to the study of the incidence and distribution of diseases and other factors relating to health.

extra-cellular matrix: the matrix of micro-fibres (collagen, elastin and amino-sugar polymers) that makes up our 'soft skeleton' and provides a structure for all our soft tissues.

familial hyperlipidaemias: inherited conditions where plasma levels of lipids such as LDL cholesterol are abnormally high. This may increase the risk of vascular disorders.

flatus: wind.

galactolipids: a family of lipid molecules that act as boundary layers and lubricants in the body.

glycogen: a polymer of glucose. Small amounts of excess glucose in the blood can be stored as glycogen, primarily in the liver.

glycolysis: the breakdown of a monosaccharide (generally glucose) into simpler components, including pyruvate.

glycosamine: an amino sugar that is the basic building block of hyaluronic acid and the amino sugar polymers in the extra-cellular matrix. The amino sugar is formed in the body by the rate-limiting enzyme glucosamine synthetase. If rates of glucosamine synthesis are too low, for example in osteoarthritis, glucosamine supplements can help to boost repairs to tissues such as cartilage.

glycosaminoglycans: complex and large molecules that, along with the fibrous proteins such as collagen and elastin, make up the extra-cellular matrix. *See* **proteoglycans**.

glycosuria: the condition where excess glucose in the blood is excreted in the urine. A tell-tale sign of diabetes.

glycosylation: a process whereby sugar molecules stick to other molecules such as proteins. When this happens, the structure and function of the protein is adversely affected. Rates of glycosylation increase when there is too much glucose (and/or other sugars) in the blood, and this is linked to tissue damage.

HDL (high density lipoprotein) cholesterol: this form of plasma cholesterol is health-promoting and cardio-protective. Formed in the liver, one of its functions is to help remove cholesterol from the linings of the arteries and return it to the liver where it can be used to form bile salts.

homocysteine: amino acid formed in the body. If there are insufficient methyl groups in your diet, homocysteine can build up to levels which are considered to be toxic. It is linked to coronary artery disease and Alzheimer's.

hyaluronic acid: a polymer of glucosamine found in the synovial fluid in joints, where it contributes cushioning and lubrication; and in the skin, where it is key to hydration.

hydration: the extent to which water is or can be held in a tissue.

hypertension: excessive blood pressure, associated with an increased risk of heart attacks and strokes, and generally caused by endothelial dysfunction.

hypoglycaemia: a condition where levels of glucose in the blood are sub-normal; it has been associated with irritability and sugar cravings.

innervate: the process whereby a nerve supplies an end organ such as a muscle.

insulin: a hormone made by the pancreas, needed to transport glucose into cells.

ions: atoms or molecules which carry one or more positive or negative electrical charges.

isoflavones: flavonoids with hormonal properties, such as genistein and daidzein. They are found in soy beans and other plants. Thought to protect against a variety of illnesses including heart disease, certain cancers and osteoporosis.

LDL cholesterol: one of the main forms of cholesterol in the blood. High levels of LDL are linked to heart disease, but this cholesterol has an important carrier function in the body. One of its main roles is to deliver valuable lipid-soluble micronutrients to the peripheral tissues (i.e. it delivers lutein that has been absorbed from the gut to the retina).

lecithin: mixed phospholipids sourced from such foods as egg yolk, which the body can use to build cell membranes, HDL cholesterol and other tissues.

liposuction: a surgical procedure whereby unwanted fat (white adipose tissue) is vacuumed out of the body.

listeria: a form of microbe involved in food poisoning in foods such as unpasteurized soft cheeses.

metabolic: a term generally used to describe the biochemistry of life.

metabolic acidosis: the blood becomes slightly more acidic – a change caused by the raised level of ketone acids (also called ketosis) which occurs when there are no carbohydrates to burn.

methyl groups: a simple group of atoms (one carbon and three hydrogen atoms) which cannot be formed in the body, and must be obtained from the diet. They are essential for DNA replication, detoxification, stress responses and other metabolic functions.

micronutrient: compound derived from the diet in milligram or microgram amounts, which are necessary for normal growth and for maintaining health. Traditionally, only vitamins and trace minerals fall into this group; more recent candidates include the flavonoids, isoflavones, carotenoids and sterols, with other new molecules waiting in the wings.

neuronal malfunction: nerves which do not work as well as they should do.

neurotransmitter: chemicals produced in the body which transfer information between nerve cells. These include acetylcholine, serotonin, dopamine and noradrenaline.

non-reactive implants: materials surgically implanted in the body (such as artificial hips) which are made out of a material, such as titanium, to which the body does not react.

omega 3 polyunsaturated fatty acids: lipids found in plant and fish oils which contain double bonds in the carbon chain. This gives them a lower melting point (so that they are liquids at room temperature), and also makes them less stable than the saturated fatty acids found, for example, in meats and dairy produce.

osteoblasts: cells that build bone.

osteocalcin: a protein made by osteoblasts, that is involved in the calcification (mineralization) of osteoid, the precursor of new bone. It requires vitamin K to start the mineralization sequence.

osteoclasts: cells that erode bone.

osteoid: a soft matrix containing protein and other microfibres, which is laid down by the bone-building osteoblast cells. Vitamin K is essential to trigger the following mineralization process, in which calcium and magnesium salts are deposited on to the osteoid, forming new bone.

oxidative: the balance between the rate of free radical formation and the body's defences against them. If there are too many free radicals and insufficient antioxidant defences, the body has a high oxidative status.

peripheral nerve damage: damage to peripheral nerves, such as occurs in diabetes, resulting in a loss of the sensations of touch and pain.

peripheral neuropathy: peripheral nerve damage.

phospholipids: molecules containing fatty acids that are produced in the liver and derived from food. They are the building blocks of cell membranes and HDL cholesterol particles.

phyto-alexins: compounds produced by plants, which they use to defend themselves against pathogens, and to some extent, predators.

phytonutrients: compounds derived from plants in our diet which are essential for maintaining health, such as carotenoids and flavonoids.

plasma lipids: fatty substances which occur in the plasma, such as LDL and HDL cholesterol.

prebiotic: formerly lumped together with dietary fibre, but now recognised as a border-line micronutrient. This is a substance available in certain foods and is required in doses of around 10 g a day in order to maintain long-term health. At these doses, prebiotics such as inulin and, more recently, ingredients such as HiMaize and Litesse, cause a profound re-organization of the bacteria that inhabit the colon, in a way that is considered to protect against colon and liver cancer.

precursor: a substance i.e. a molecule, from which another molecule or tissue is formed.

probiotic: healthy bacteria consumed in fermented milk products or as supplements, which may be useful in treating certain types of diarrhoea, colitis and pouchitis. This approach is not very effective at changing gut bacterial populations.

protein denaturation: changes in the structure of proteins which lead to a loss of the function of that protein. Glycosylation causes denaturation, as does heat (which is why egg whites turn solid when cooked) and extremes of pH.

proteoglycans: highly complex and extremely large molecules that, along with the fibrous proteins such as collagen and elastin, make up the extra-cellular matrix. *See glycosaminoglycans.*

Q10: the rate-limiting co-factor in oxidative phosphorylation, an antioxidant, and a mitochondrial protector. Broadly, this means that Q10 is essential for energy formation.

RDA: recommended daily allowance.

receptor: in cell biology, a structure on the surface of a cell (or inside a cell) that selectively receives and binds a specific substance, and subsequently triggers a cellular or physiological response.

renal failure: a condition in which the kidneys' functions have become compromised. Mild renal failure or impairment is often difficult to detect. More severe renal failure may necessitate dialysis or a renal transplant.

salicylates: compounds found in many plant foods which have anti-inflammatory effects in the body. A synthetic product, acetylsalicylate, is the active compound in aspirin and has been linked to a reduced risk of thrombus and colo-rectal cancer.

salmonella: a genus (group) of bacteria, many of which can cause food poisoning.

saturated fats: fats which are found predominantly in meats and dairy foods. They have a high melting point so are generally solid or semi-solid at room temperature.

simple carbs: sugars such as fructose, glucose or sucrose.

statins: drugs used to lower levels of LDL cholesterol in the bloodstream. Depending on the individual, they may have severe side-effects.

symbiotic (functional foods definition): a product which combines prebiotics with probiotics.

T-cells: immune cells involved in defence against various pathogens. Targeted by HIV.

thrombus: a clot in a blood vessel, which may, depending on the size and site of the affected vessel, cause mild to life-threatening symptoms.

tocopherols/tocotrienols: a group of important fat-soluble antioxidants derived from plant foods. These include gamma tocopherol and D-alpha tocopherol, which is used in old-fashioned supplements. Mixed tocopherols and tocotrienols offer better protection.

toxins: poisons.

triglycerides: fatty molecules which occur in the diet, and which are also found in the bloodstream. Levels tend to rise after a meal; sustained high levels are considered to increase the risk of heart disease.

type A malnutrition: the near-absence of a micronutrient, leading to a deficiency disease such as the severe lack of vitamin C, which causes scurvy. Type A malnutrition is often accompanied by calorie shortage, and generally only found in developing countries.

type B malnutrition: multiple micronutrient depletion, often accompanied by calorie excess, which leads to metabolic imbalance and catabolic dominance. This in turn lays the foundations for most, if not all, of the major chronic degenerative diseases. This type of malnutrition is prevalent in the developed world.

vascular disease: disease affecting the blood vessels.

vasodilators: compounds which make constricted blood vessels dilate, leading to a reduction in blood pressure.

Further Resources

Clayton, P, *Health Defence* (2nd ed.) (Bucks, Accelerated Learning systems, 2004)

Websites

- For more information on pharmaco-nutrition and health maintenance, *see*: www.healthdefence.com
- For information on brown adipose tissue and how to regulate it, *see*: www.adrenaline.org

Notes and References

Introduction: The Clayton Plan – A New Way to Health

1. National Audit Office (February, 2004) 'Tackling Obesity In England', National Audit Office Report
2. Cancer Research UK, (9 September, 2004 – last update), 'Breast Cancer', available: http://www.cancerresearchuk.org/aboutcancer/specificcancers/breastcancer
3. Better Health Channel, (March 2004 – last update), 'Smoking and Eye Disease', available: http://www.betterhealth.vic.gov.au/bhcv2/bhcarticles.nsf/pages/Smoking_and_eye_disease
4. Shifrin, T. (8 September, 2004) 'Coalition launches manifesto for chronically ill', *Guardian*
5. Starfield, B. et al. (2000) *JMA*, vol. 284 (4), pp483–5

Part 1: Atkins Examined
2 Health Concerns

1. Foster, D. G. et al. (2003) 'A Randomized Trial of a Low-Carbohydrate Diet for Obesity', *New England Journal of Medicine*, vol. 348 (21), pp2082–90
2. Smith, M. (21 January, 2004 – last update), 'Atkins Diet goes on a Diet Review', available: http://content.health.msn.com/content/article/79/96354
3. Gerber, R.T. et al. (1999) 'Cholesterol-independent endothelial dysfunction in virgin and pregnant rats fed a diet high in saturated fat', *The Journal of Physiology*, vol. 517 (2), pp607–16
   See also:
   Fuentes, F. et al. (2001) 'Mediterranean and low-fat diets improve endothelial function in hypercholesterolemic men', *Annals of Internal Medicine*, vol. 134 (12), pp1115–19
4. Reddy, S.T. et al. (2002) 'Effect of low-carbohydrate high-protein diets on acid-base balance, stone-forming propensity, and calcium metabolism', *American Journal of Kidney Diseases* vol. 40, pp265–74
5. Please note that this is the author's overview of the literature – there is no single reference that would clearly support this statement.
6. Fernandez, F., Hill, M. J. (1990) in Kritchevsky, D., Bonfield, C., Anderson, J. W. (eds), *Dietary Fiber: Chemistry, Physiology, and Health Effects*, Plenum Publishing Corporation, pp417–29

See also:
Alberts, D. S. et al (2003) 'Fecal Bile Acid Concentrations in a Subpopulation of the Wheat Bran Fiber Colon Polyp Trial', *Cancer Epidemiology Biomarkers & Prevention*, vol. 12, pp197–200

7. Mizutani T. and Mitsuoka, T. (1980) 'Inhibitory effect of some intestinal bacteria on liver tumorigenesis in gnotobiotic C3H/He male mice', *Cancer Letters*, vol. 11, pp89–95
    See also:
    Mizutani T. and Mitsouka, T. (1979) *Journal of National Cancer Institute*, vol. 63, pp1365–70
    Reddy, S. and Rivenson, B.A. (1993) *Cancer Research*, vol. 53, pp3914–18
    Koo, M. and Rao, A. V. (1991) *Nutritional Research Reviews*, vol.51, pp137–46

3 But Fruit and Veg *Are* Good For You!

1. Krinsky, N. I. et al. (2003) 'Biologic mechanisms of the protective role of lutein and zeaxanthin in the eye', *Annual Review of Nutrition*, vol.23, pp171–201
    See also:
    Gale, C. R., Hall, N. F. et al. (2003) 'Lutein and zeaxanthin status and risk of age-related macular degeneration', *Investigative Ophthalmology and Visual Science*, vol. 44 (6), pp2461–5

2. Kohlmeier, L. et al. (1997) 'Lycopene and myocardial infarction risk in the EURAMIC Study', *American Journal of Epidemiology*, vol. 146 (8), pp618–26
    See also:
    Rissanen, T.H. et al. (2003) 'Serum lycopene concentrations and carotid atherosclerosis: the Kuopio Ischaemic Heart Disease Risk Factor Study', *The American Journal of Clinical Nutrition*, vol. 77, pp133–8
    Sesso, H. et al. (2004) 'Plasma lycopene, other carotenoids, and retinol and the risk of cardiovascular disease in women', *The American Journal of Clinical Nutrition* vol. 79, pp47–53

3. Dwyer, J. H. et al. (2001) 'Oxygenated Carotenoid Lutein and Progression of Early Atherosclerosis: The Los Angeles Atherosclerosis Study', *Circulation*, vol. 103, pp2922–7
    See also:
    Makita, H., Ohnishi, M., Mori, H., Satoh, K. and Hara, A. (1995) 'Chemoprevention of Rat Oral Carcinogenesis by Naturally Occurring Xanthophylls, Astaxanthin and Canthaxanthin', *Cancer Research*, vol. 55, pp4059–464

4. Dwyer, J. H., (2001) *Circulation*, vol. 103, pp2922–7
    See also:
    Levy, J. et al. (1995) *Nutrition & Cancer*, vol. 24 pp257–67 and. Kohlmeier, L. et al. (1997) 'Lycopene and myocardial infarction risk in the EURAMIC Study', *American Journal of Epidemiology*, vol. 146, pp618–26

5. Kohlmeier, L. et al. (1997) 'Lycopene and myocardial infarction risk in the EURAMIC Study', *American Journal of Epidemiology*, vol. 146 (8), pp618–26
    See also:
    Rissanen, T.H. et al. (2003) 'Serum lycopene concentrations and carotid atherosclerosis: the Kuopio Ischaemic Heart Disease Risk Factor Study', *The American Journal of Clinical Nutrition* vol. 77, pp133–8

6. Sesso, H. et al. (2004) 'Plasma lycopene, other carotenoids, and retinol and the risk of cardiovascular disease in women', *The American Journal of Clinical Nutrition*, vol. 79, pp47–53
    Landrum, J. T., Bone, R. A., Joa, J., Kilburn, M. D., Moore, L. L. and Sprague, K. E. (1997) 'A One Year Study of the Macular Pigment: The Effect of 140 Days of a Lutein Supplement', *Experimental Eye Research*, vol.65 (1), pp57–62

7. Fung, T. T., Stampfer, M. J., Mason, J. A. E., Rexrode, K. M., Willett, W. C., and

Hu, F. B. (2004) 'Prospective Study of Major Dietary Patterns and Stroke Risk in Women', *Stroke*, vol. 35, pp2014–19

8. Chen, I., McDougal, A., Wang, F. and Safe, S. (1998) 'Aryl hydrocarbon receptor-mediated antiestrogenic and antitumorigenic activity of diindolylmethane', *Carcinogenesis*, vol. 19, pp1631–9
   See also:
   Meng, Q. et al. (2000) *Journal of Molecular Medicine*, vol. 78, pp155–65
   Hudson, E. A. et al. (1998) *Biochemical Society Transactions*, vol. 26, S370

9. Myers, L., Bouic, P., (1998) *Proceedings of the 26th Annual Congressional Physiology Society SA*
   See also:
   Bouic. P. et al. (1999) *International Journal of Sports Medicine*, vol. 20, pp258–62

10. Breytenbach, U. et al. (2001) *Cell Biology International*, vol. 25, pp43–9
    See also:
    Bouic, P. et al. (2001) *South African Medical Journal*, vol. 91, pp848–50

4 The Good Carbs

1. Pierre, F., Perrin, P., Champ, M., Bonnet, F., Meflah, K., Menanteau, J. (1997) 'Short-chain Fructo-oligosaccharides Reduce the Occurrence of Colon Tumors and Develop Gut-associated Lymphoid Tissue in Min Mice', *Cancer Research*, vol. 5 (2), pp225–8

2. Hata, Y et al. (1983) 'The effect of fructo-oligosaccharides (Neosugar) on lipidemia', *Geriatic Medicine*, vol. 21, pp156–67

3. Bjorck, I. and Elmstahl, H. L. (2003) 'The glycaemic index: importance of dietary fibre and other food properties', *Proceedings of the Nutrition Society*, vol. 62 (1), pp201–6

4. Remesy, C. et al.(1992) in T. F. Schweizer and C. A. Edwards, *Dietary Fibre – A Component of Food: Nutritional Function in Health and Disease*, Springer-Verlag, London, pp137–50
   See also:
   Wright, R. S., Anderson, J. W. and Bridges, S. R. (1990) 'Propionate inhibits hapatocyte lipid synthesis', *Proceedings of the Society for Experimental Biology and Medicine*, vol. 195, pp26–9

5. Govers, M. J. A. P., Gannon, N. J., Dunshea, F. R., Gibson, P. R. and Muir, J. G. (1999) 'Wheat Bran Affects the Site of Fermentation of Resistant Starch and Luminal Indexes Related to Colon Cancer Risk: A Study in Pigs', *Gut*, vol. 45, pp840–7
   See also:
   Buddington, R. K., Williams, C. H., Chen, S. C. and Witherly, S. A. (1996) 'Dietary Supplement of Neosugar Alters the Fecal Flora and Decreases Activities of Some Reductive Enzymes in Human Subjects', *The American Journal of Clinical Nutrition*, 63, pp706–16

Part 2: The Clayton Plan
5 The Clayton Plan Step 1: How to Eat

1. Giovannucci, E. (1999) 'Tomatoes, tomato-based products, lycopene, and cancer: review of the epidemiologic literature', *Journal of National Cancer Institute*, vol. 91 (15), pp1331
   See also:
   Giovannucci, E. et al. (2002) 'A prospective study of tomato products, lycopene, and prostate cancer risk', *Journal of National Cancer Institute*, vol. 94 (5), pp391–8

2. The Free Dictionary.com, (2004 – last update), 'Sulphite', available: http://encyclopedia.thefreedictionary.com/Sulphites
3. Food and Behaviour Research, (2004 – last update), 'About FAB Research', available: http://www.fabresearch.org/view_item.aspx?item_id=3
4. Which? News Release Archive, (September 2004 – last update), 'The Raw Deal from Supermarket Fruit and Veg', available: http://www.which.net/media/pr/jun04/which/fruitveg.html

8 The Clayton Plan for Exercise

1. The United States Department of Health and Human Services, (29 December 2003 – last update), 'Physical Activity Fundamental to Preventing Disease', available: http://aspe.hhs.gov/health/reports/physicalactivity/index.shtml
2. Ibid
3. Ibid
4. There is no published data on this subject as of yet as the research is very new and the work ongoing.

Part 3: Fighting Disease with the Clayton Plan
9 Vascular Disease, Type 2 Diabetes and the Dementias

1. Simopoulos, A. P. (2002) 'Omega-3 fatty acids in inflammation and autoimmune diseases', *Journal of the American College of Nutrition*, vol. 21(6), pp495–505
2. Linseisen, J. and Wolfram, G. (1998) 'Absorption of Cholesterol Oxidation Products from Ordinary Foodstuff in Humans', *Annals of Nutrition and Metabolism*, vol.42, pp221–30
3. Sensi, M. et al. (1995) 'Role of advanced glycation end-products (AGE) in late diabetic complications', *Diabetes Research and Clinical Practice*, vol. 1, pp9–17
See also:
Peppa, M. et al. (2003) 'Glucose, advanced glycation end products, and diabetes complications: what is new and what works – Council's Voice', *Clinical Diabetes*
4. Pegel, K (1997) *South African Journal of Science*, vol. 93, pp263–8
See also:
Bouic, P. J. D. et al, (1996) *International Journal Immunopharm* vol. 18, pp693–700
5. Xu, Y. et al. (1998) *Hematophol Mol Hematol*, vol. 11, pp49–62
See also:
Ferreira, J. et al. (1994) *Res Comm Mol Path Pharmacol*, vol.94, pp147–55
6. The American Heart Association, (2004 – last update), 'Phytochemicals and Cardiovascular Disease', available: http://www.americanheart.org/presenter.jhtml?identifier=4722
7. Omar, M. A. and Wilson, J. P. (2002) *Reactions 1*, vol.4-4 (1), pp1
See also:
Folzenlogen, D. (2001) *Journal of Clinical Rheumatology*,vol. 7, pp340–5
Jackson, P. R. et al. (2001) *British Journal of Clinical Pharmacology*, vol. 52, pp439–46
8. The American Heart Association, (2004 – last update), 'Elevated homocysteine in heart patients linked with higher stroke risk', available: http://www.americanheart.org/presenter.jhtml?identifier=3008854
9. Karpinnen, H. and Mervaala, E.(1996) *Journal of Human Hypertension*,vol. 10 (1), pp57–61
See also:
Gelijnse, J. M. et al.(1994) *British Medical Journal*, vol.309, pp436–40
10. O'Donnell, C. D. (1998) 'A short salt synopsis', *Prepared Foods*

11. Hodgson, J. M. and Wahlqvist, M. L. (1993)'Nutrition and health of Victorian Aborigines (Kooris)', *Asia Pacific Journal of Clinical Nutrition*, vol. 2 (1), pp 43–57
12. Media.McDonalds.com, (2004 – last update), 'Media Statement: McDonald's Response to "Super Size Me" Movie', available: http://www.media.mcdonalds. com/secured/news/pressreleases/2004/Press_Release04292004.html
13. International Diabetes Monitor Archives, (August 2004 – last update), 'Oxidative stress and Type 2 diabetes', available: http://www.medforum.nl/idm/leading.htm
14. Schönlau, F. and Rohdewald, P. (2001) 'Pycnogenl® for diabetic retinopathy', *International Ophthalmology*, vol 24 (3), pp161–71
    See also:
    Spadea, L. and Balestrazzi, E. (2001) *Phytotherapy Research*, vol. 15 (3), pp219–23
15. This product is widely available for purchase on the web. Simply type 'Mannose' into your browser for more details.
16. Schonlau, F. and Rohdewald, P. (2001) 'Pycnogenol for diabetic retinopathy. A review', *International Ophthalmology*,vol.24(3), pp161–71
    See also:
    Varma, D.(1986) 'Inhibition of aldose reductase by flavonoids: Possible attenuation of diabetic complications', *Progress in Clinical Biology Research*, vol. 213, pp343–58
    Lanthony, P. and Cosson, J. P. (1988) 'The course of color vision in early diabetic retinopathy treated with Ginkgo biloba extract. A preliminary double-blind versus placebo study', *Journal of French Ophtalmology*, vol. 11, pp671–4 (in French)
17. AD2000 Collaborative Group (2004) 'Long-term donepezil treatment in 565 patients with Alzheimer's disease (AD2000): randomised double-blind trial', *Lancet*, vol. 363, pp2105–15
18. Zhuang H. et al. (2003) 'Potential mechanism by which resveratrol, a red wine constituent, protects neurons', *Annals of the New York Academy of Sciences*, vol. 993, pp276–86; discussion 287–8
    See also:
    Savaskan, E. et al.(2003) 'Red wine ingredient resveratrol protects from beta-amyloid neurotoxicity', *Gerontology*, vol. 49, pp380–3
    Pace-Asciak, C. R. et al. (1996) 'Wines and grape juices as modulators of platelet aggregation in healthy human subjects', *Clinica Chimica Acta*, vol. 246, pp163–82
    Meng, X. et al. (2004) 'Urinary and plasma levels of resveratrol and quercetin in humans, mice, and rats after ingestion of pure compounds and grape juice', *Journal of Agricultural and Food Chemistry*, vol. 52, pp935–42
    Commenges, D. et al. (2000) 'Intake of flavonoids and risk of dementia', *European Journal of Epidemiology*, vol. 16, pp357–63
    Engelhart, M. J. et al. (2002) 'Dietary intake of antioxidants and risk of Alzheimer disease', *Journal of the American Medical Association*, vol. 287, pp3223–9
    Rinaldi, P et al.(2003) 'Plasma antioxidants are similarly depleted in mild cognitive impairment and in Alzheimer's disease', *Neurobiology and Aging*, vol. 24, pp915–19
    Zandi, P. P et al. (2004) 'Reduced risk of Alzheimer disease in users of antioxidant vitamin supplements: the Cache County Study', *Archives of Neurology*, vol. 61, pp82–8
19. Deans, S. G. et al. (2002) 'Experimental Gerontology' in Knook and Hofeker (eds) (1994) *Aspects of Ageing & Disease,* 9th Symposium
    See also:
    Facultas Wien Hagen, T. M. et al. (2002) 'Feeding acetyl-L-carnitine and lipoic acid to old rats significantly improves metabolic function while decreasing oxidative stress', *Proceedings of the National Academy of Sciences*, vol. 99, pp1870–5
    Liu, J. et al. (2002) 'Memory loss in old rats is associated with brain mitochondrial decay and RNA/DNA oxidation: Partial reversal by feeding acetyl-L-carnitine

and/or R-alpha-lipoic acid', *Proceedings of the National Academy of Sciences*, vol. 99, pp2356–61

Liu, J et al. (2002) 'Age-associated mitochondrial oxidative decay: improvement of carnitine acetyltransferase substrate-binding affinity and activity in brain by feeding old rats acetyl-L-carnitine and/or R-alpha-lipoic acid', *Proceedings of the National Academy of Sciences*, vol.99, pp1876–81

10 Joints, Bones, Skin and Cancer: The Regeneration Game

1. Reginster, J. Y. et al. (2001) *The Lancet*, vol. 357, pp251–56000
   See also:
   D'Ambrosio, E. et al. (1981) *Pharmatherapeutica*, vol. 2 (8), pp504–8
2. Glucosamine can no longer be sold as a supplement in Norway as it is now classified as a medicine.
3. Shearer, M. J. (1995) *The Lancet*, vol. 345, pp229–34
   See also:
   Loveridge, N., (1993) *Proceedings of the Nutrition Society*, vol.52, pp49–55
4. Rossouw, J. E. et al. (2002) 'Risks and benefits of estrogen plus progestin in healthy postmenopausal women. Principal results from the Women's Health Initiative randomized controlled trial', *Journal of the American Medical Association*, vol. 288 (3), pp321–33
   See also:
   Manson J.E. et al. (2003) 'Estrogen plus progestin and the risk of coronary heart disease', *New England Journal of Medicine*, vol. 349 (6), pp523–34
   Wassertheir-Smoller, S. (2003) 'Effect of estrogen plus progestin on stroke in post-mentopausal women. The Women's Health Initiative: A randomized trial', *Journal of the American Medical Association*, vol. 289 (20), pp2673–84

Part 4: New Directions in Total Health and Well-being
11 New Ways to Stop Smoking

1. Buck, D. and Morgan, A. (2001) *European Journal of Public Health*, vol.11 (2), pp211–17
   See also:
   Wisbord, K. et al. (2000) *Clinical Obstetrics and Gynecology*, vol. 96 (6), pp967–71
   Daughton, D. M. et al. (1999) *Preventive Medicine*, vol. 28 (2), pp113–18
2. Bollinger, C. T. et al. (2000) *The Medical Journal of Australia*, vol. 172, pp279–83
3. Pauly, J.L. et al. (2000) 'Safe Cigarette Alternatives? Industry Critics Say "Not Yet"', *Journal of the National Cancer Institute*, vol. 92 (8), pp660
4. Tobacco Free Kids, (2004 – last update), 'New Scientific Study Contradicts R.J. Reynolds' Claims That Eclipse is a "Reduced-Risk" Cigarette', available: http://tobaccofreekids.org/Script/DisplayPressRelease.php3?Display=305

13 Natural Viagra

1. Chew, K. K. et al. (2000) *The Medical Journal of Australia*, vol. 172, pp279–83
2. This information comes from unpublished research carried out at the University of Beijing.
3. Personal communication report of a conversation between the author and Dr Purvis.
4. UCLA Health Sciences, (2004 – last update), 'Soy Phytoestrogens May Ease Menopausal Symptoms', available: http://www.healthcare.ucla.edu/vital-signs/article-display?article_id=279

14 New Ways to Burn Fat

1. Huttunen, P. J. et al. (1981) 'Occurrence of brown adipose tissue in outdoor workers', *European Journal of Applied Physiology & Occupational Physiology*, vol. 46 (4), pp339–46
2. Bray, G. (1980) 'Blame it all on brown fat now', *Medical News*, vol. 243 (20), pp1983–4
3. Krief, S. et al (1993) 'Tissue distribution of β_3-adrenergic receptormRNA in man', *Journal Clinical Investigation*, vol. 91, pp344–9
4. Himms-Hagen, J. et al. (2000) 'Multilocular fat cells in WAT of CL-316243-treated rats derive directly from white adipocytes', *American Journal of Physiology*, vol. 279 (3), pp670–81
5. Lean, M. E. J. (1989) 'Brown adipose tissue in humans', *Proceedings of the Nutrition Society*, vol. 48, pp243–56
   See also:
   Garruti, G. and Ricquier, D. (1992) 'Analysis of uncoupling protein and its mRNA in adipose tissue deposits of adult humans', *Internal Journal of Obesity*, vol. 16, pp383–90
6. Kakkar, V. (1993) 'Try the cold water treatment', *The European*, vol. 155, pp1
   See also:
   Kakkar, V. (1993) 'Why I had to publish now', *The European*, vol. 155, pp7
   Kakkar, V. (1993) 'How to take the waters', *The European*, vol. 155, pp6
   Kakkar, V. et al. (1993) 'Brown adipose tissue thermogenesis as physiological strategy for adaption', *Japanese Journal of Physiology*, vol. 43, pp117–39
7. Dauncey, M. J. (1981) 'Influence of mild cold on 24hr energy expenditure, resting metabolism and diet induced thermogenesis', *British Journal of Nutrition*, vol. 45, pp257–67
8. Kates, A. and Himms-Hagen, J. (1992) 'Effects of cold acclimatization and fasting on thyroxine 5-deiodinase in brown adipose tissue of OB/OB mice', *Proceedings of the Society For Experimental Biology and Medicine*, vol. 200 (4), pp495–501
9. Heaton, J. M. (1972) 'The distribution of brown adipose tissue in the human', *Journal of Anatomy*, vol. 112 (1), pp35–9

Chapter 14 is very in-depth, and as such a general reference for the whole chapter is necessary:
http://64.233.183.104/search?q=cache:7FqCB8qhej0J:www.sportsci.org/encyc/drafts/Brown_adipose.doc+Huttunen+children+brown+adipose+tissue&hl=en

Index